ERRATA

Page 49, line 36 for "ten" read "hundred"

Page 133, line 5, for "reorganised" read "recognised"

To Bryony and Pat
with the best wishes
of the author.
Christmas 1972.
R Hughes Parry.

UNDER THE CHERRY TREE

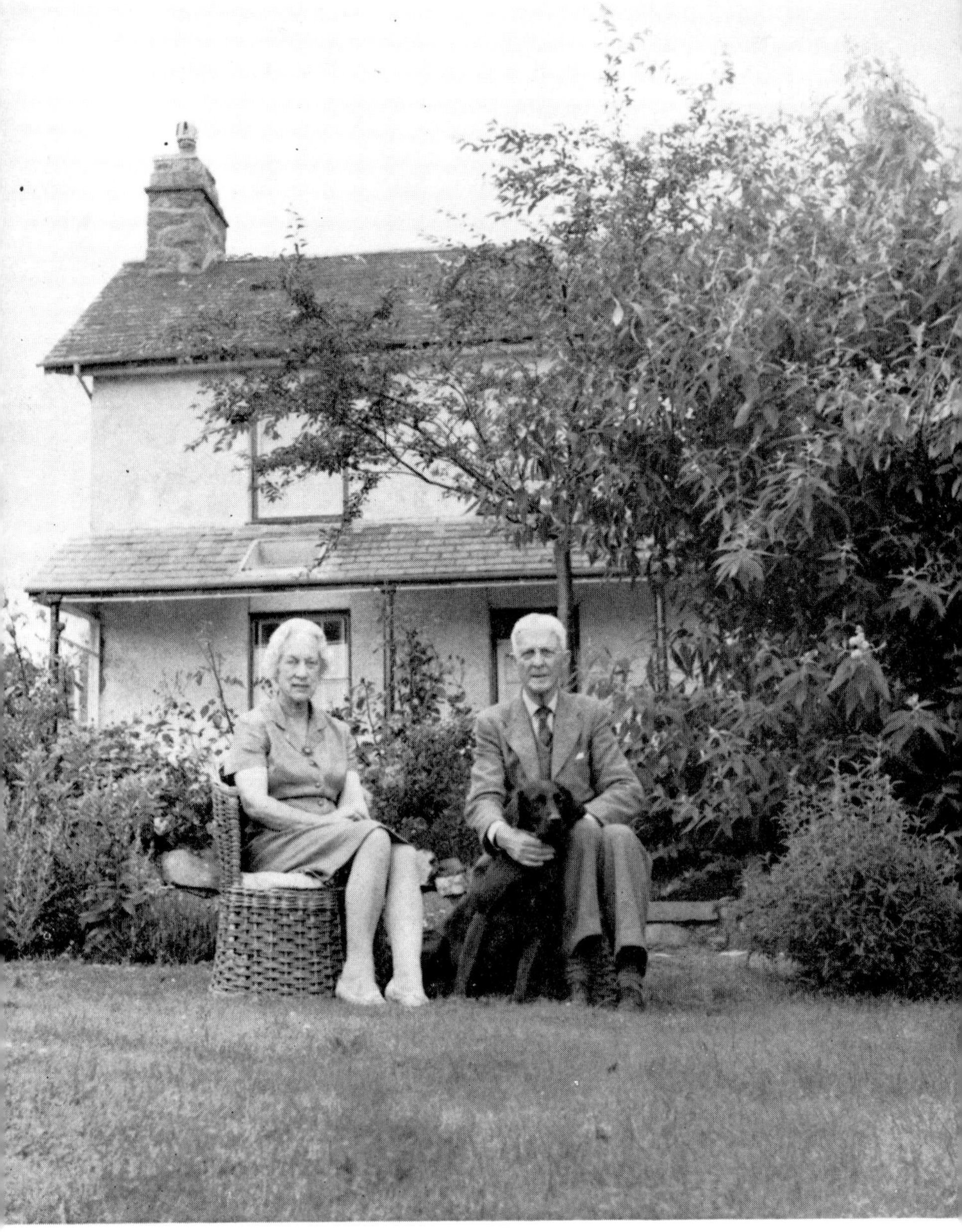

"Under the Cherry Tree" (1969)

Under The Cherry Tree

by

ROBERT HUGHES PARRY

GOMERIAN PRESS
LLANDYSUL
1969

First Impression, November 1969

PRINTED IN WALES BY
J. D. LEWIS AND SONS LTD.
GOMERIAN PRESS, LLANDYSUL

Dedication

In gratitude
to Joan for her help and encouragement for forty five years
and to the memory of my Father and Mother
who made all this possible

FOREWORD

I AM glad to commend UNDER THE CHERRY TREE. It is a lively account of the experiences of a man who has been Doctor, General Practitioner and Chief Medical Officer. Just as interesting are the author's comments on contemporary happenings and his occasional excursions into other countries, the United States, Persia, Greece.

I first met Dr. R. H. Parry when I was a young parson and heard him lecture on the housing situation in Bristol. His graphic descriptions of the appalling Slum Conditions in the city filled me with a desire to help to create housing facilities suitable for family life. I stood for election to the Bristol Council and subsequently became Chairman of the Health Committee with Dr. Parry as the Chief Medical Officer. I recall these years with happiness and I believe that his vision and guidance helped all of us on the Committee to embark upon some valuable pioneering efforts. Indeed it is as a pioneer in the municipal health service that I think of Dr. Parry. He had the ability to see several steps ahead, but, unlike some visionaries, he had the administrative wisdom to know how the goal could be reached.

It is fourteen years since he left Bristol, but his name is still remembered. And, although he would be the first to say that many have contributed to the excellence of the health services in the city, they are in part his own testimonial and witness.

MERVYN SOUTHWARK

Bishop's House
38 Tooting Bec Gardens,
Streatham,
London, S.W.16.

INTRODUCTION

YEARS ago, when I was a resident physician to the General Post Office in the City of London, I occupied a small furnished flat within a stone's throw of St. Paul's Cathedral. Many other young doctors occupied that same flat before me and several had left more than one mark of their tastes in the matter of pictures and such like. I have often wondered who could have left a picture on the front of an old calendar hanging on the wall of the bedroom. It was of a pretty Japanese girl in a large straw hat sitting in the shade of a cherry tree with an abundance of cherries all around her on the ground and on the tree.

Underneath was the caption :

> "In the hum of the market there's money,
> under the cherry tree there's rest".

I was then in the "hum of the market" but maybe the seed of the idea of being able to sit "under the cherry tree" was sown then. Now that day has arrived, I hope in these pages to live once again some of the interesting events that have occurred in a long and happy life.

Cefniwrch,
Criccieth.

1969.

CONTENTS

PLATES

CHAPTER I

EARLY LIFE AND STUDENT DAYS

I WAS born in 1895 and still retain certain clear impressions of life at the turn of the century. I remember my father and mother as they were then—my father was tall, about six foot, and proportionately built ; a strong athletic type, and, as I now realise, very good-looking. He had a dark, trimmed moustache and hair parted in the middle. His hearty laugh could be heard and recognised from afar and he was always ready to enjoy a joke and to play one on anybody. He was rather short-tempered and hasty in those days but always most kind and generous and mellowed much in his later years. Although an excellent public speaker in Welsh he was a bad linguist and spoke only broken English, and was shy withal. On many occasions in those days this proved a great handicap to him. He did nor read widely —except, of course, his daily English Language paper. Having started with the *Daily Mail* during the South African War he kept it up for many years, and it was his favourite paper to the end of his days.

My mother was also tall. Slightly above average and slim, with long hair shading to auburn, she had penetrating, beautiful blue eyes and a fresh complexion. I was told many times by the old women of the village that she was the most beautiful girl they had ever seen. She was very capable, could sing well and was most energetic. Although she tolerated and almost encouraged my father's jokes and ' leg-pulls,' I never thought she had a very keen sense of humour. She was a great practical Christian and many a poor person in the district had cause to be grateful for her kindness. It was a wonderful home in which to be brought up with the dominating influence and the disciplinarian being my mother, as of course it should be. Rarely did my father join in because he was more easy-going but, when he did, we all knew and recognised it !

My first home, which I remember well was a stone-built farmhouse called *Uwchlaw'rffynon* on the southern slopes of the Rivals in Caernarvonshire. It was not the original house because there were a few remains of an old house some fifty yards away which had been demolished and the newer one erected sometime in the middle of the

19th century. There were a few trees to protect the house from the east and the west. Some of my happiest memories to this day are of the sound of the trees during the gales that often came our way. Even today I am still fascinated by the sound of the wind in the trees. From the front windows of the house we looked down to the sea and along the coast of Cardigan Bay halfway to St. David's. To the left, behind the lower hills, were the high mountains of Snowdonia. To the left still—eastwards—was a gap between the lower hills and the Rivals to the north, and, as the crow flew, this gap led straight onto the Menai Straits and the Isle of Anglesey. This view was to be seen from a higher vantage point behind the house. Westwards, to the right, was a hill which hid away the plain in the centre of the Lleyn peninsula where, later on, we were to move to live. The house stood by itself, a quarter of a mile from its nearest neighbour which was another farmhouse. A couple more hundred yards was the village at the bottom of the valley in full view of our house.

My father John was the third son of John Parry of Penllwyn, near Pwllheli. He had spent much of his youth with his grandfather, Dafydd Hughes at Clogwyn, a few miles from his parents' home. My mother, Ann, was the eldest child of Henry Hughes of Cwmcorcyn which faced Uwchlaw'rffynon on the opposite slope of the valley. where her ancestors had owned and farmed this estate for at least a thousand years. Before her marriage she was living with her grandfather, Robert Hughes at Uwchlaw'rffynon. Dafydd Hughes and Robert Hughes were brothers so my father and mother were second cousins. My parents started married life on this farm with Robert Hughes who was then eighty years old and he remained in their care till his death a few years later.

About this time my mother's parents decided, together with some families from the neighbourhood, to emigrate to the middle west of the United States of America. All the children went with their parents except my mother but one sister returned later.

I have very happy memories of this home on the side of the Rivals at the foot of Tre Ceiri, the mountain peak. I recollect most vividly crawling, as a young child of five or six, to the mouths of large holes in the ground covered with slabs of slate, to drop stones between the slates, and listen for the sound of them reaching the water. It was great fun in those days, but sometime later it came back to me with something of a panic, because a dog had fallen into one of these and there was no hope of his recovery. The same feeling must have possessed my father for it did not take him very long to fill the holes with stones and soil. These holes were the result of my great-grandfather's venture into the field of geology. In company with his wealthy land-owner he had traversed the area with a divining rod looking for precious metal and, where the rod indicated, they had dug deep. As far as I know no precious metal was found.

I have vague recollections of heavy snowstorms when all the hedges completely disappeared, and all hands on the farm were mustered to dig out the sheep and to feed them. I have a similar, not-too-clear memory of the preparation of the meat for the family and staff. A bullock had to be killed once a year to supply the beef, which had to be salted on the big kitchen table, and also pigs several times a year and sheep even more often. I recollect an old fellow, usually known as "Butch," bringing a large pig in a cart to be killed on the farm—obviously on this occasion we did not have a suitable one ourselves. "Butch," as usual, had called at the various taverns on the way and, when he came out of the last one of them at our village, the pig was making a lot of noise and continued to do so. He lost his temper and, taking his knife, he "stuck" the pig in the cart until the blood flowed freely, and left a track all the way to our house. My father was intensely annoyed, but knew too well that a drunken man is hardly ever reasonable. Such conduct would create a good deal of consternation today, and the authorities would soon step in—but this happened nearly seventy years ago.

Those slaughtering days on the farm were also feast days, and we all looked forward to the roasting and the eating that followed. One dish in particular attracted us—"brwas" (pronounced brooas). This was made in a very large wooden bowl with white bread filling the bottom. Then specially prepared oatmeal cake was crushed and the bowl filled up after which boiling beef or mutton broth was poured over and the whole allowed to soak well and to cool ready to eat. The staff would then sit round the wooden bowl, select the nearest spot, and eat away with their spoons. Whenever we could we joined in, but mother would not permit us if she found out, for we had a small bowl each. I always imagined it was never as good in a small bowl.

The picture I have of the farm kitchen stands out very clearly in my memory. It was a rectangular room, thirty five feet long, with two long windows. Along one side was a large table, scrubbed white, with two large cupboards, into each of which went a sack of flour, and a set of drawers in between. On the other side of the room were two old Welsh dressers, one filled with willow pattern plates and the other with pewter plates, both sets of which were of various sizes. Between the two dressers was the old brass-faced grandfather clock with its friendly familiar tick and strikes, and a shining brass preserving pan at the base. Hanging from the wall were brass bed warmers, and, in the corner, the old oak arm-chair with the date 1673 carved on the back in large numbers. I have that in my possession now. From the hooks in the ceiling were hung large pieces of bacon. The mantlepiece had rows of brass candlesticks. What a wonderful sight it was at the end of the week, the farm work over, to see the kitchen spotlessly clean ! The womenfolk of today would not tolerate the work that would be involved in keeping a kitchen of this size in the state I now remember. Why should they ? But what they miss ! In an oven next to the fire baking of bread occurred once a week, and the oven was also heated up on Saturdays for the Sunday meals.

Many a pleasant hour did I spend in this kitchen with its roaring wood fire which was sometimes of peat with its pleasant smell. There were two other large sitting rooms and there was often a fire in one of these, but we liked the kitchen best for the life of "our world" was centred there.

I well remember the birth of my younger brother, Ceiri. I was then five and a half years old. The morning of the first day after his birth I was called up to the bedroom to see my mother and the baby, and was then packed off by myself to inform our neighbour on an adjacent farm, some three quarters of a mile away.

Ultimately we were a family of five children and I was the middle one. The eldest, Catherine, or Cats as we called her, was six years older than myself. Dafydd was three years older than I and my young sister, Primrose was born five years after Ceiri and did not arrive on the scene until we have moved to Penllwyn.

There was another event that impressed me very much when I was about six years old. My parents and baby brother had gone out to supper to a farm some three or four miles away. We three other children were comfortably installed in the front room in the charge of the maid. Late in the evening there was considerable consternation outside with people calling out, and the sound of rattling buckets.

The maid ventured out and found that all the men were back and others were with them, rushing to try and put out a fire which had taken hold of a huge rick of corn. It had been a very fine harvest and all the corn had been made into one big rick whilst waiting for the threshing machine to come. It was not insured and there was little doubt that this was incendiarism, for the fire had been started in several places. Very little was saved because the rick was well alight before the fire was discovered, and it was so combustible after the dry harvest. It was not possible to find sufficient evidence to implicate anyone, but my parents were satisfied that they knew the culprit. My mother always believed in some unseen power behind the scene and this power, she believed, would actively intervene when injustice was done, and even punish the culprit. Since then I have often seen injustice done, but it has not always followed as mother would have it. But I heard her say often afterwards that the winter following the fire was a most successful farming time for us ! In spite of shortage of feeding, the animals seemed to have made a special effort to help the farm economy ! On the other hand the family of the supposed culprit started its way down the slippery slope and, if the guess was right, never could it be truer to say that the sins of the father were visited on the children. However, my mother argued further and insisted that the fact that the culprit's family did suffer was evidence of the father's guilt. I wonder ? It does make one wonder for the ways of nature are strange.

I well remember my first journey to school where I went when I was nearly five years old. It was a Board school in the village, and the headmaster, John Roberts, an upright little man with a waxed moustache, had a large family of daughters and two sons. One of the daughters sang very well and for practice she was required, at times, to come and sing before the school. We thought very highly of the headmaster, but I think we might have shown more gratitude to him in his old age. If he had had financial and other support he would have made a success of his school. Built of stone it was big, clumsy and high-ceilinged. It was L-shaped, and the wing could be shut off with doors to form a junior class-room. I was brought in by my brother and handed over to the care of the pupil teacher in charge of the junior class. She was the eldest daughter of the headmaster, and could not have been more than seventeen or eighteen years old at that time. Over fifty years later I was sent by the British Information Services to speak at the Waldorf Astoria to the Cymrodorion Society of New York at the celebration of St David's Day. The first person I met was my pupil-teacher, now an elderly lady and an American citizen, as also were two of her sisters.

I do not remember much of my school days in this village school. Nothing in particular happened and I am sure it was not unpleasant otherwise I would remember.

I have a vague recollection of repercussions from the South African War, of catastrophies and victories, and of heroic names like Buller and Lord Roberts. About the same time there were local elections when my father, to the disgust of his uncle, succeeded in knocking him out from being a Guardian of the Poor, and a District Councillor. This perhaps was my father's first election to the District Council where he continued for nearly fifty years, and was Chairman of the Board of Guardians for the last twelve years of its existence.

When I was seven years of age I became the proud possessor of a penknife. How this came about I cannot now recollect, but the instrument, 'made in Sheffield,' must have cost six pennies and was much appreciated. I soon learnt how to keep it sharp by using the 'stones' which the men on the farm used to sharpen their tools. My chief use of the knife was to make whilstles with cuttings from sycamore, and it was just as well perhaps that there was plenty of space in the fields so that the noise could hardly cause annoyance to anyone. Then, of course, I could make 'tops,' although there was little opportunity to play this game in those days of untarred roads and unconcreted paths. Soon after possessing this wonderful tool I was sent on an errand to the village. It was a Saturday afternoon and I was returning slowly along the road using my knife on a piece of wood when a tall working-man came marching along and caught up me. Now I knew about this man although he had never spoken to me. He worked at a granite quarry at Trevor some three or four miles down the valley near the sea. On Saturday afternoons, like many others of his fellow workers, he used to go home, returning on Sunday evening to his lodging near the quarry. His home at Nefyn was about nine miles from Trevor where he worked and the road led above our house along the side of the mountain. It was a difficult road with two or three steep hills and since bicycles were not common in those days, and there was no public transport, he had to walk home and back. We knew him as "Twm JaJa", and he could not be mistaken for anyone else for he had a hair lip and cleft palate which affected his speech considerably. When he came up to me he stopped and said, "Have you a penknife ?" With a feeling of general numbness stirred slightly by curiosity and without a word I handed him my knife. He sat on the side of the road, took his heavy boot off his foot, stripped off a thick woollen sock, which had been heavily darned in the heel and, with my knife, cut off the heel of the sock. Then, putting his heeless sock back on his foot, followed by his boot, he muttered his "Thanks" and stepped off again. What a vivid impression that little incident made on my young mind ! My father had a more amusing story that than one to tell of "Twm JaJa". One Sunday evening, on his way back to his lodings, he had come the best part of six miles and on the road above our home, some five hundred yards away, he came into the full face of a gale that was blowing through the gap between the mountains from the north east. He had been trying to light his pipe as he was going along, but his only hope was by crouching by the hedge for some shelter and turning his back to the wind. Having succeeded at last, he straightened up and trudged along. It was just as he reached home again that he realised he had not turned round after lighting his pipe, so that it meant an extra twelve miles walk for him that night !

I well remember, too, another Twm who had a little pony and a light cart, and who from time to time used to come along the mountain road shouting in Welsh, "Herrings—herrings fresh" in a wonderful baritone voice. There was a story abroad that whilst shouting thus one day Twm dislocated his jaw and had to go at once to the local doctor to be treated. The story went that when his jaw snapped back into its place he uttered the word "fresh" to complete his shout !

About 1905, when I was nearly ten years of age, my parents decided to move to my father's old home—a farm lower down the plain, about two miles from the south coast of the Lleyn Peninsula which would give us a warmer climate and be more convenient for the town of Pwllheli and its school. Our new home was about half a mile from the nearest village, Efailnewydd, but the village children had to walk a distance of at least a mile, past our home, to the village of Llannor to attend the church school. The excitement of changing homes lasted a short while only and for the next five or six years I do not think many things stand out very clearly in my mind. Mostly I remember how I missed my old home—my walk up to the mountain on autumn mornings before going to school to remove the flat stone from the hole in the mountain wall, and the march down to the farm followed by the sheep. That was now finished. Now I was nearer to people with very little chance of being by myself tramping the fields and the mountain side.

I do remember, in my first home, regretting very much not being one of the village lads, so that I could roam the village as one of them, visit the cobbler's shop and the blacksmith and see and hear what was done and said at these centres of village life. It is also true that when the weather was inclement and I was confined indoors either in the house or in the farm buildings, I could have done with companionship, although I would have appreciated a workshop even more. I hardly remember playing with my elder brother Dafydd, and sister Cats, and even now cannot imagine what they found to do. My other brother Ceiri was six years younger so that he was of little use to me—in fact he was a considerable nuisance when it became my resposnibility to keep an eye on him—which task I evaded whenever I possibly could. To be left alone as I was to organise my own sport and pleasure does breed a spirit of independence and self confidence which can be either a help or a hindrance later on in life. I have often wondered whether or not I could possibly have suffered in silence the discipline of a boarding school after being allowed so much freedom. Of course, "nothing is so good but it may be abused,"—so with freedom, so with discipline. I shall forever be grateful that I was brought up in the midst of plenty of food and with ample clothing. Although the value of these treasures was not appreciated at the time, there is no doubt at all that they were to stand me in good stead both during my years of rapid growth and later. I am now old enough and have seen enough of the world to appreciate that a child during his early school life needs plenty of food, exercise and rest, and, may I add, freedom, under happy conditions. Far too much stress is laid on education and too little on training.

I could not have been more than six years of age and yet one particular incident has remained with me as a very vivid picture all my life. It all happened because I caught a cold which was followed by pneumonia. I was put to bed, in the nursing care of my wonderful mother and the occasional supervision of the old family doctor who lived eight miles away. In his day the doctor was reckoned to be an able general practitioner and in later years I was able to confirm this for he was in active practice until he was well in his eighties and died at the noble age of 96. We as a family had great confidence in him—had he not attended at least one of my great grandfathers ! When in his 93rd year he insisted on my newly-qualified son scanning his chest with the old doctor's own old wooden stethoscope—that he might know "what healthy old age was like."

One sunny day in Spring I was let out of the house, wrapped well up against the cold. I was permitted to go and watch the men dragging stones in sledges from the mountain to build a wall on the farm. When a hundred yards or so from the mountain quarry I met a loaded sledge with a white mare led by one of the men whose name I have forgotten. I could take you to that spot now. He was delighted to see me and as a welcome picked me up and placed me on top of the loose stones on the sledge. I never got a grip before the white horse was off and I slithered down between his legs. The man never saw me and the noise of the sledge drowned my cries. My only hope was to race on all fours and get to the side but I made no progress on the rough ground. With a mighty, desperate effort I threw my arms round the mare's hind leg and she realized there was something wrong and succeeded in stopping the skidding sledge. The man looked up and then down, saw me and rescue came. I can't remember being scared or crying, but for many years after I remember waking up at night, shouting and gripping hard at the nearest object. I promised that I would never mention it to my parents and never did. Why should I ? It was just an accident and I was not worried. The philosophy of a child ! I don't remember being nearer death than that, as far as I know. But then, who does know ?

An event that impressed itself very much upon my memory occurred about the same time as this last escapade. I remember sitting proudly between my brother and sister in the back of the trap whilst my father and mother with my baby brother in her arms were in the front. A fast black pony, Sally, and a grand-looking rubber-tyred trap were, of course, what I admired most at that moment. I had very much in mind the story my father had brought back from the market town one Wednesday a few weeks before. He had ridden the pony to town and left it in the stables of the Crown hotel. When he called round early in the afternoon to see if it was alright he found to his dismay that it was gone. With mounting anger he went to the street wondering what to do, when he saw Sally being led along by a stranger. The man was soon, and without much ceremony, dispossessed and it took him a while to impress upon my father that he represented the British Army and was purchasing horses for the South African War. Of course, no money could buy Sally and I am sure that after that narrow escape she was more valuable than ever in our eyes.

On that day—it might have been a Sunday, we were on our way to see and hear Evan Roberts, the young university student and famous revivalist, who was holding an open-air meeting at the village of Abererch. I remember clearly standing amidst the thousands and hearing this fine young man with a shock of curly black hair and penetrating silver voice standing up on a platform and addressing the crowd. He called on all sinners to repent and, as my father remarked afterwards, directed his attention particularly to those who tried to shelter from his attention behind trees. My father's admiration for him was increased by this, because it showed he had lots of common sense—what would now be called a knowledge of human psychology. On many occasions since I have had to address meetings on St. David's Day, usually an after-dinner address, and I have never been able to resist mentioning the impression Evan Roberts left on me as a child. I am told that St. David was a man with a most impressive personality and a voice which could be heard from afar, above the commotion created by "protesters" of those days. Of course, both men must have had a message which was worth hearing.

I remember something of the revival at the beginning of the century as it affected the village and village life—the personalities who were lifted out of the gutter and remained model villagers, and others who drifted back when the old temptations of drinking and rough living threw them again into poverty and degradation. The tuneful hymns sung with vigour and feeling still stick in my memory. From this remote distance and with limited experience of the occasion, I am still deeply impressed with the amount of influence for good it brought to the community where it occurred. I cannot visualise the return of a religious revival, but I do sincerely regret that narrow, bigotted religious oppression by the chapel leaders at the time never permitted true Christianity to develop. We are suffering today as the result.

From the time the family moved into the new home, where my father's ancestors had lived, until I left the county school, no very strong impressions were left on my mind. I can recollect a good deal of the day routine work—cycle to school, lessons, cycle back about three miles, help with the farm work, changeable weather. I can remember the times well but there were no very deep impressions. Rather, the time was filled with eating, going to school, coming back and playing. The summer time when we all took a part in the harvesting was particularly pleasant and it brought with it a feeling of fitness and 'joie de vivre'. It was during this time that my mother told everybody that I wanted to be a doctor. I don't remember telling anyone but I accepted it as my own decision. I don't even remember being enamoured with the idea but, at the same time, I never thought of any other profession for I was going to be a doctor and I musn't change my mind. In school I was not very good at Science, but I was good at Mathematics and I enjoyed History very much. All the same, I was going to be a doctor one day. My brother Dafydd was a very good mathematician and chemist but weak in History, yet he became a lawyer. I just don't know how such things come about. Indeed, today I often think that I would have been much happier as a lawyer, and yet—I wonder ! I was always interested in people. Business, as far as I could see, was to get as much out of people as possible and the legal profession was out for discipline—"according to the law". The church was concerned with reprimanding and threatening. But at least there was a chance to study people and maybe to help them if I became a doctor, or so I thought at the time. The doctors into whose hands I fell in those days were kindly and fatherly and did indeed possess the bedside manner which has been so notable by its absence in so many of the doctors I have met since. It is quite possible I did not rebel against the decision, be it mine or my parents, to become a doctor, because of this. My dear mother was always concerned about my health and I have no doubt she thought that if I qualified I would look after my health better but that, of course, does not follow at all.

Clear pictures of some of the people of that time remain with me to this day. There was the headmaster of the local Church school, Gethin Jones. Strangely enough he was Welsh but could not speak Welsh and yet there was hardly a child in the school who understood English, much less spoke the language at home. But we all liked him and he took a lot of trouble to try and understand us. He insisted that I should try an entrance scholarship to the County School—I was then ten years old. Under his guidance I came seventh on the list and as there were only three scholarships I was not successful, but I entered the County School the following year. Forty years later this same headmaster returned to the neighbourhood by which time he was Rural Dean and a Canon of Gloucester Cathedral. When he heard I was at Bristol he left a message with my brother Ceiri that he wished me to call and have tea with him and gave his address. When, eventually, I turned up at his vicarage at Kempley with my wife and a friend in the friend's Rolls Royce, the vicar was entertaining friends to tea in the garden at Kempley. Of course, he had not the least idea who I was and was most embarassed when I reminded him that he had invited me to tea. "Not today, did I ?" said he, most worried, "Not today" I replied, "but is today inconvenient ?" "Oh no, not at all". I tried to direct his attention to the old vicarage and the garden but I could see he was more anxious to find out who I was. At last I took him to meet my wife and friend and then he suddenly realised who I was. Result—the nearest thing to a hiding I ever got from my old headmaster ! His son, Eric, whom I remember as a young lad, had by now followed in his father's footsteps and become vicar of his father's former parish of Dymock in Gloucestershire and Canon of the Cathedral. He also became Queen's Chaplain and gained great honours during the war.

I was successful with my work at school because I was the lucky possessor of that faculty which in the modern world is essential to academic success—' examination aptitude '. This gave me the Chairman's scholarship after my brother Dafydd had left school and finished with it.

Sometimes during my schooldays I heard, amongst others, Lloyd George speak at political meetings. After one of these meetings another schoolboy and myself fought our way to up the platform and insisted on shaking hands with him. He was just surprised, put his hand on each of our shoulders, shook hands and said nothing. I also heard the cultured Sir Rufus Isaacs and was most impressed with his style rather than what he said.

At the age of sixteen I matriculated, London University, and, immediately after the examination, with a plea of ill health, vanished to some relations on a remote mountain farm on Cennin mountain. It was a most wonderful holiday of four lovely months in the summer of 1912 and it did build up my strength. I spent most of the time by myself wandering along the mountain side or chasing sheep. When the holiday was over I found myself at Aberystwyth University

College—I was then only seventeen years of age and should have returned to school for at least another two years.

Today I realise I was completely oblivious to what was happening in the world outside during those years. The suffering, the poverty, international quarrels, political intrigues—they all took place outside my life and I don't remember paying any attention to newspapers. But I do remember with some satisfaction writing an essay in the London Matric exam on "International Peace" and declaring confidently for a Council of Nations to be formed to stop petty quarrelling and intrigue amongst the nations of the world. But this was not a subject that public opinion was yet ready for and it needed at least two more wars to make people realise that this was something worth considering and bringing into being.

I entered the Middlesex Hospital Medical School in October 1914 as a second year student.

Those were hard days for university students whose parents did not have plenty of money to support them because there were no government grants to help them. I had to remember that I was a farmer's son, the middle of five children and only my sister Cats had left the nest. My brother, Dafydd, was soon to be in the army for four years and when he returned there was no grant available to him because he had a degree in Economics before entering the army on his way to obtain a law degree. If that happened today there would be at least a demonstration in Downing Street ! Even when I qualified in 1916 my first appointment of house surgeon at the Middlesex Hospital carried with it no salary at all, only full board and lodging and two pounds ten shillings a half year washing allowance.

No account of my student days in London would be complete without a brief account of a visit for a week-end during my first year in London of William Hughes, the senior deacon of our village chapel. He was well-known in the district of my home as the owner-worker of a threshing machine which was moved about the countryside by teams of horses from farm to farm. It seems that he had come to London to look for a new machine and he was accompanied by his son Roger, who assisted him in the threshing season. I decided to take time off and keep them company on a sight-seeing tour of London. The old gentleman was then in his early seventies and a more open-minded man I have never met. He insisted either on walking or travelling on the top of one of the old red 'buses—preferably the former if that were practicable. He was not impressed with big buildings nor with Buckingham Palace but insisted on stopping at Hyde Park Corner for ten minutes to count the motor cars coming out of the Park. He wondered what it would be like in fifty years ! He stopped in the Strand, stamped his feet on the paving-stones and said "I do admire their pavements". We went to the theatre one evening and this he thoroughly enjoyed although he confessed he did not understand all that was said since Welsh was his usual language, but he could see nothing wicked in it as he had been led to believe at home. One Sunday morning we were walking up Whitehall and struggling up the incline was a lorry full of coal drawn by one horse. William Hughes noticed that the horse was hardly making any progress up the slippery road. He threw his coat and hat to his son and said "A horse is a horse wherever it is" and went to the rescue by turning the wheel of the cart. He came back to us and said "It has a load of a ton and a half. At home we never expect one horse to draw more than fifteen hundredweights" !

How refreshing to have a clear open mind expressing its views on the world around us.

As a raw medical student at the Middlesex I was attached as a surgical dresser to Sir John Bland Sutton and soon became aware that I was in the presence of a great man. He was then at the height of his fame—senior surgeon to the Middlesex Hospital and President of the Royal College of Surgeons. He was a pioneer of abdominal surgery and, as pioneers do today, suffered much from destructive criticism. In the main this comes from three directions—from those who want to see life standing still ; from jealous colleagues ; and, worst of all, from publicists whose only hope of fame is to bite the lion. He was truly a great surgeon, a great writer and a great lecturer and in all these spheres he showed the capacity for taking infinite care.

He was a small, rather plain man with a big nose and pale complexion, but with black penetrating lively eyes. He was never tired of saying how much he owed to his parents. His father was a butcher in Pentonville and had taught him how to wield a knife. His mother for her part, taught him the Bible and he made full use of the knowledge in his profession. Above all he was human, approachable, humble and gentle with a keen sense of humour and the reflection from these simple qualities made his greatmess stand out.

He used to tell of a woman patient, seriously ill in hospital. He thought she had a chance if operated upon and told her to think about it for a day or two. When he returned to the ward two days later she was reading the Bible and, when he glanced over her shoulder and saw it open at a certain chapter in the book of Jeremiah the prophet of doom, he knew the answer to the operation would be "no" and so it was !

One day when he came for his round he took me by the arm and said "I am not so full of energy this morning—one of those society receptions. What I like most about those parties is when our guests have all departed and I can take my wife by the arm down to the kitchen and make ourselves a cup of tea. All the same, my boy, if you think you can be as happy as I am, marry a wealthy woman."

On his way up the ladder, when he was plain "Mr", he was called to see a certain Earl who was seriously ill. It was decided to operate in the castle that day. The Countess interviewed him in the library and after the operation he reported to her in the library again. "And now," said the Countess, "you will want some refreshment. The butler will take care of you." The butler took him to his pantry and gave him a most acceptable cup of tea and two boiled eggs." "Believe me, my boy," he said, "each of those two eggs cost the lady one hundred guineas !"

What a privilege for a young Welsh boy from a mountain farm in Caernarvonshire to study at his feet.

What should have been the happiest of my student days were marred by the Great War. Those of us who were well on with our studies had been asked to stay and complete the course because we would be more useful later on. Considerable responsibilities were cast upon us because of a shortage of qualified staff and whilst working for my final exam I served for three months in 1917 as house-surgeon at the East Suffolk and Ipswich Hospital which was used largely for the treatment of war casualties.

Strange events stand out in the mind—whether or not they happen to be important. On one occasion I was receiving a convoy of casualties from France into my ward in the early hours of the morning when I noticed a face that I thought I knew. Later, whilst doing a round to see if all the patients were comfortable, I came to this man. He was an ordinary "Tommy" suffering from trench fever. I spoke to him but he just stared and made no reply but as I was turning my back to go to the next bed realisation suddenly dawned upon me and I turned round and addressed him in Welsh. He became so excited, he nearly jumped out of bed and then explained his strange behaviour. He was a monoglot Welshman who understood little and spoke no English. He had been posted to an English battalion and had spent most of his army service in the trenches in France where language was not important ! One night in the trenches he thought he saw a former employer but when he spoke to him he received no reply and then the vision vanished. Now he thought he was experiencing the same thing again. I applied for his transfer to a hospital in Wales where he could understand what was said to him and this was soon granted. Some forty years later three men called to see me here at Cefniwrch, having driven thirty miles by car. The old man had brought his two sons to see me, having told them of his experience when he was a soldier, and to thank me once again for my help. Who said that memory is short ? When I was a boy I knew him as a farm-labourer on my sister's farm.

Another little episode of my student days took place one Sunday morning when I went to a Welsh Chapel in North London and an elderly gentleman came to shake hands and welcome us after the service. I answered his questions about myself and suddenly he said "Would you come and join me for Sunday dinner ?" What hungry medical student in those days before grants could refuse such an offer ! I went with him and found myself in a palatial house in Harley Street. When the meal was over he took me to his study and there he revealed his interest in me. He was Dr. Lloyd Williams, consultant dentist at the Royal Dental hospital, Leicester Square and when he was a small boy my great-grandfather, who was a friend of his father, used to visit his home near Caernarvon and he gave me a most interesting account of my great-gandfather and his hobbies.

I did well enough at the Medical School to be awarded a Broderip scholarship in clinical medicine and surgery, and the Lyell scholarship and gold medal in Surgery which helped me to obtain several resident posts at the Middlesex Hospital—House-Surgeon to Mr. Sampson Handley, Casualty Medical Officer under Dr. R. A. Young (later Sir Robert Young) and Casualty Surgical Officer under Mr. Webb Johnson (later Lord Webb Johnson). Yes, they were happy days, with plenty of work and responsibility but, above all, with "chiefs" who could not but be admired and indeed almost worshipped.

Talk of Mao's Flu in the 1960's brought back to my memory the 1918 infleunza epidemic in this country. When the 'flu broke out towards the end of 1918 I was resident Medical Officer at the Middlesex Hospital and my duties consisted of receiving all medical casualties from 9 a.m. to 5 p.m. There was never a more hopeless task than mine during the epidemic. People by the score walked or were brought in from the West End of London to Casualty Department of the hospital. They had been well when they started out in the morning and had suddenly collapsed in the street. Their cyanosed colour was ghastly and really I did little more during the day time than direct the traffic to the wards—mostly to the emergency wards and some even to the mortuary. Of course, I went down myself just in time to miss the armistice but I soon recovered. I do hope we shall never see anything like that again. That epidemic was worldwide and caused more deaths and disablement than the first War itself—in India alone it was estimated that 6 million people died. In England and Wales where no no such mortality had ever been recorded before nor has been since about 150,000 people died. The strange feature of this epidemic was that it affected so many people in the prime of life, the largest proportion of deaths being in those under 45 years, whereas we were, and indeed are still, accustomed to think of influenza as a disease that affects and kills mostly in old age. Why was it so severe in 1918-19? We were, at the time, well satisfied with the idea that the catastrophe of the World War which had lasted so long had drained our physical resources and affected severely our mental health through our worries and this had lowered our resistance. I wonder what modern epidemologists would say to such an 'old-fashioned' explanation.

Of course, we had not heard of antibiotics in those days. Many years later, during the Second World War, as a member of the Medical Advisory Council of the Nuffield Provincial Hospitals Trust, I was privileged to be present when the possibility of such a discovery was brought to our notice.

It came as a request from a young bacteriologist at Oxford, Howard Florey. He had been worried at the thought of seeing thousands of our soldiers dying with gas gangrene of their open wounds, as had happened in the First World War. He had searched the literature and found a reference to an observation several years before by Alexander Fleming, a bacteriologist at St. Mary's Hospital in London, that a mould had destroyed bacteria in vitro cultures. He thought there were great possibilities and he wanted a grant to follow it up and investigate further. Of course, we all most willingly supported the idea, and a grant was given from the Nuffield Fund.

A few months later, sitting next to Hugh Cairns, the famous brain-surgeon, at dinner, I was thrilled to hear of his experience with the experimental use of penicillin on some of his patients. He summarised it by saying that most of his surgical work on the brain would not be required if further experience proved his experience so far with penicillin to be correct.

But the early penicillin was not the pure painless drug that we are accustomed to use today. My wife reminds me of this fact for she was one of the early victims of a painful injection for a streptococcal infection of the face. After two injections she insisted she would rather die than have a third ! So I persuaded her it was the injector rather than the injection and I volunteered to inject but it was equally painful if not worse ! By good luck the three injections were sufficient but she still remembers the pain.

A few years before, Sulphonamides had been discovered and their mode of use in treatment worked out by my friend Lionel Whitby at the Middlesex Hospital. I saw some remarkable recoveries from bacterial infection cured by their use, including a cellulitis in the fore-arm of my eldest daughter. Oh, what would I not have given to have had these drugs at my disposal as a casualty officer or when in general practice !

An interesting period of my life was when I was engaged for three years from 1921 to 1923 on cancer research at the Middlesex Hospital. My post was Assistant to the Professor of Experimental Pathology and the Professor was Lazarus Barlow. When I look back I do not think I appreciated as much as I should the ability and the kindness of my chief. But then what young man does ? I wish, however, I had shown a little more admiration which would have been so acceptable and could have done nothing but good.

I had an idea about cancer, and I still have it but do not know how to prove it that cancer is "body repair out of control". However, this is not a treatise on cancer and there is much to be said for this point-of-view, but not on this occasion. I learned much during those three years. I learned to think and had time to do so.

It was while I was working on this research that I met my future wife—that fortunate event which has meant so much in my life. She was then Joan Williams, a final year medical student at the Royal Free Hospital.

One day my former chief, W. Sampson Handley, called to see me in the laboratory. He came purposely to warn me that I must not remain a "lab" man. I had been his house-surgeon and he thought my true calling was amongst people and not amongst animals and dead tissues in the "lab". This turned my life right round. At that time another old friend, Percy Stocks the world famous statistician, was sharing my room in the laboratory and I told him what Handley had said and he strongly advised me to take on public health. He suggested Bristol, where he himself had served, as a fine city in which to start. I thought hard, discussed it with my fiancee, and so started another life.

Many Welsh men and women have spent most, if not all of their working days outside their own country. A general criticism has been levelled against us that we could have made a greater contribution to Welsh life and Welsh culture if we had returned to serve Wales in our own line. That, I fear, is true, but it has not been altogether our faults. I would like to quote two amusing incidents that occurred in my own life to illustrate my point and I am sure many of the criticised 'exiles' could give other examples.

Just at the time when I was deciding to take up public health work an advertisement appeared for a School Medical Officer in Carmarthenshire and I applied as I was qualified with D.P.H. and had plenty of clinical experience. A friend of mine, Alwyn Lloyd, living in Burry Port, heard of my application and advised me to canvass but I pointed out that this was specifically prohibited. He declared, however, that it was only put in to encourage canvassing, which sounded strange to me! I asked a farmer uncle, D. H. Davies of Rorsedd, a County Councillor in my native county, to come with me. In the course of our canvassing we called on a well-known farmer who was on the appointing committee and walked round his farm. If I remember rightly he was the Committee's Vice-Chairman. Then my uncle broached the subject of our visit. The councillor was most sympathetic but declared quite honestly that qualifications and merit were not to be considered. Two local boys, one a Calvanist and one a Baptist, were applying and one of these was to be appointed depending on the relative strength of the denominations on the Council. The few Independents could be ignored. I was not even on the short list and the Calvinist was appointed. A few weeks later I was appointed to a post in Bristol out of sixty-three applicants.

Many years later I was approached about the possibility of my being considered for the post of Chief Medical Officer for Wales. I stated my terms without ambiguity but at the same time expressed my feelings that I would much rather not undertake the task although I was quite prepared to help as far as possible. Two days later I was told it was "not on". It would appear that I was "persona non grata" as what was wanted was a Medical Officer who would do as he was told by the administrators ! Besides, to separate Wales from Whitehall would reduce the opportunity for promotion which existed for officials working in a region, Wales being then a region of England. Lest we blame politicians for everything we should remember that self-interest also dominates the lives of many individuals in every sphere of life.

CHAPTER II

GENERAL PRACTICE IN PWLLHELI, 1925-27

After one year as an assistant School Medical Officer in Bristol I decided I could not continue with the monotonous and unexciting work. After all, I had spent some years as a resident at the Middlesex Hospital, a year in the Royal Air Force and three years in cancer research and to try, day in day out, to carry out routine examinations as a school medical officer was more than I could stand. So my wife, who had by now qualified as a doctor, and I decided to settle down in general practice in my home town, in a house in the centre of the town. The three years we spent in general practice in Pwllheli were perhaps the most exciting period of our lives. It was exciting because we were young and receptive and we learned much about how people lived and what made for a happy and useful life.

The other doctors in the town, of whom there were four, were old and tired and although our conduct was a little unethical in those days it had good results at once. Two of the doctors appointed young assistants with a view to partnership. I had the advantage that my ancestors had been for several hundred years prominent and, I think, reasonably respected in the county. My father was Vice-Chairman of the Magistrates and Chairman of the Board of Guardians which he served for nearly fifty years. I realised that factors like these counted far more with people than qualifications which they did not understand.

One wealthy old lady, in her eighties, sent for me and asked me to look after her for the rest of her days. She confessed to me one day that the reason she was so anxious to have me as her doctor was because my great grandfather had given her half a crown when she was a little girl. Bribery and corruption of course—but he did not know! She was a wonderful patient, delicate and sensitive, but responsive to persuasion. On one occasion I went away for a week and left her to the care of my wife and another doctor. When I returned she was in an exhausted condition as she had not been able to sleep and every effort with sleeping draughts had only made her worse. I sat by her bedside, made her a little tasty potion, mostly water, told her to go to sleep and kept my hand on her forehead. In five minutes she was fast asleep and remained so all night. She died two years later and afterwards her son came to me and said he was glad she had died before I left the practice. What a compliment ! This was a great lesson to me and I sincerely wish that our medical students today could have the chance of learning about the opportunities for service that rest with the general practitioners in what is often an art rather than a science ! How often does a patient enter hospital, have his systems examined and found to be normal but is discharged still a sick man ? The man is a whole, not a collection of systems. When the National Health Service Act was under consideration, I exerted all the influence I had to try and persuade those in authority that general practice should first of all be organised or reorganised and supported for therein lies our hope for a healthy nation. After all, the need for hospital means that prevention has failed.

An old solicitor in the town—he, too, was in his eighties and was one of the County people—called on us one day and asked me to keep an eye on him. He warned me that he would not be a lucrative client because he was never ill. He also declared, "You may think my boy that you are well-qualified. That may be so but I would like you to know that I am asking you to look after me because, when I was a young lad, your great grandfather took me out with him to canvas for an election—in the Conservative cause and don't you forget that ! We visited another great grandfather of yours and I have never had such delicious boiled beef in my life before or since !" A couple of years later his wife called me to see him. He was President of the District Golfing Union for the year and had been away for a week. When he came back he had every sign of cardiac failure and I took him to his room to examine him on his bed. When that was over, I stood up and said to him something on these lines. "Sir—your heart apex beat is three inches down and out, your liver is considerably enlarged, your feet and legs are pitting with dropsy and you have heart failure. Now listen to me—if you had continued with your usual habits of a bottle of rum every three days, pink gin well-diluted when thirsty and your usual wines with your lunch and dinner, you would probably be good for another ten years. I suppose you have been mixing everything during the last week ?" "Yes—they had no rum !" "Now don't you be a damn fool like this again to harm yourself and worry your wife". "Have you finished ?" "Yes". "Who the hell are you talking to ? This old world owes me nothing !"

I am told that is how he died some years later but I was away and did not see him.

Yes, "roots" are very important. Not only are they important to the doctor but also to the patient. I knew many of the old and young families around the town and countryside. I knew their family history and I had some idea of their will to live which was a great help both to them and to me. I have mentioned elsewhere what a blessing came with the sulphonamides and the antibiotics. No one can estimate how many lives have been saved by their use. They are the greatest boon since Jenner discovered vaccination and helped to wipe out smallpox from our country.

As in most walks of life coincidence also plays its part in the life of the general practitioner. One Saturday night I was reading the *British Medical Journal* in front of the fire in the sitting-room. I had just read an article by a pathologist on "hanging" in which he defined the difference between suffocation and strangulation when the door-bell sounded. I was wanted down in the town where the policemen had just cut down a suicide. At least I was perfectly sure of my diagnosis—on a subject on which I had known nothing before I read the article.

I have said that we settled down in a very convenient house in the centre of the town of Pwllheli. Just on the edge of the town, up a little hill, was a lovely Georgian house in its own grounds. My wife and I went to see it and we fell for it at once. Our friends warned us that it was much less convenient from the "business" point of view but no argument influenced us and we rented the house and settled down. Our first child, our eldest daughter, was born there and we decided to call her Ann after my mother. One day a week or so later an old blind man who had been born and brought up in the town, John Williams by name, commonly known as Jack-one-Eye, who had been born and brought up in the town where he had been a coalmerchant, called on me with his boy guide. He congratulated us on our daughter and asked her name. "Ann" said I. "It is as it should be. I was afraid I would not be in time," he replied. And then he told this story :—

Many years previously, he said, probably more than a hundred and fifty, the land on which our house stood was merely a small hillock without any buildings round it. It overlooked the harbour and in the days of which he spoke the sea came much nearer than at the time he was telling me his story. The land, apparently, had been owned by a farmer-timber merchant who lived in a small mansion a quarter of a mile away and his timberyard stood at the bottom of this hill. One morning after a heavy storm which had lasted several days this man stood looking out to sea and saw a ship stranded on the rocks outside the harbour. With an eye to business, and knowing the coast and its dangers, he had the ship surveyed and the report came back that it was a Scandinavian sailing vessel called *Anna*. She was carrying a cargo of Spanish mahogany timber, and there was a good chance of salvaging the cargo at least. He at once bought the cargo and, having salvaged it successfully, proceeded to build a house on this site. The doors, stairs, and even the windows were made of Spanish mahogany and became known locally as "Mahogany Hall". He then moved into his new hill-top house to live and his only child, a girl, was born there and named Anna after the Scandinavian ship. As far as our story teller had been able to find out ours was the only child to have been born there since. The house had changed hands a few times but this merchant, he said, had been an ancestor of mine.

We were able to verify this story later, and on removing the old paint work discovered that even his statement about the mahogany window frames was true.

I thanked him for the information, and when we handed the practice over to our successors—a newly married couple—their first child was a daughter and they called her Ann for their own family reasons. Other families have lived there since but we have refrained from further enquiries lest the "magic chain" be broken !

There have been many repercussions of our days in practice but I shall mention only two. A few years ago I went for a game of golf with my son to a local golf club and as we drove up to the parking ground, a powerful-looking young man came up to us. The conversation went something like this (in Welsh of course). "Are you the doctor ?" "Yes." "I owe you, sir, more than I can ever repay. Do you remember looking after a family with four boys living in this village at Morfa Nefyn ?" "Yes, I do". "Well, I was the youngest and the puniest of the family—always ill and I could never join my brothers in their sport. You were called in again one day for something or other. I was then about nine years old and very downhearted. You must have realised that I was dreadfully depressed. You stood me up on the bed, patted me all over my body and then made a little speech. "You come from a healthy family, look at your brothers. You think you are the exception. Not a bit of it ! Your turn is coming later and you will be as big as if not bigger than any of them. Patience my boy ; wait for it.' I am bigger and stronger and have had a healthy life so far. Thank you. From that day I never looked back."

The other occasion was also on the golf links in the days when a person of moderate means could afford a caddy. It was competition day in the local club and I was on holiday. We went off the first tee after a respectable drive and chatting away with the caddy I enquired if he was a local man. "Yes." "Where do you live ?" " . . . Terrace". "What number ?" "Ten." "Then your father was the fisherman ?" "Yes". "How old are you ?" "Twenty one." 'Well I brought you into the world didn't I ?" "Yes sir." But I remembered that I hadn't for he was on the floor when I arrived ! I missed my next shot and lost the hole !

The local doctors were all personalities and had their followers. We were a very friendly group always ready to help one another. One country doctor who looked after a group of villages about seven miles away was a particularly amusing character. He was later followed by his son who was not quite up to the old man's standard. Many good stories are told of the senior Dr. Rowlands. Discussions had taken place both locally and at Government level about extending the railways through South Caernarvonshire to Nefyn and the doctor was very anxious to see this done for the convenience of the people. Mr. John Burns in the Campbell Bannerman Ministry came down to see the doctor, the countryside and the possibility of extensions, no doubt influenced by Lloyd George. They spent the evening discussing the problem but not to the satisfaction of the doctor. With dawn next morning the doctor aroused his guest who protested vigorously at the unearthly hour. "Not at all", said the doctor, "you will want all this time because your train goes at 10.30 and you have only a little over four hours to breakfast and walk seven miles to the station." "I must have a cab." "We have no cabs in this village and my old nag is lame. Now what about the train and spoiling the scenery ?" But he never got the railway.

As my wife and I were driving in our little open Morris two-seater through the street he stepped smartly off the pavement to stop the car. "Congratulations on your second child," he said. "Turning out children like pills, aren't you ?" Our final score was only four which was hardly worth such a compliment.

He oscillated between drinking and abstinence and during one of the latter periods was elected Superintendent of the Sunday School. In the Committee after the meeting one Sunday the coal-merchant protested that the doctor never delivered his own prayer as was the custom in the chapel but made the congregation join him in the Lord's Prayer. After listening patiently the doctor turned to the members of the Committee and said, "What's wrong with the Lord's Prayer? Which would you rather, His or the Coal-Merchant's?" This character has long since passed on but for a long while happy memories of his great kindness and good work remained throughout the land. Now, alas, these memories have nearly all dimmed or disappeared and the world goes on.

In my days there was a unique opportunity for the general practitioner to know his people and he was nearer to them than the minister or parish priest or lawyer. He helped them to make up their minds about many personal problems such as wills, family quarrels and disputes. He knew and was interested in their family budgets and it wasn't difficult to calculate—5/- a week in Poor Law Relief and £1 a week to a good workman with four or five children! Even so, the children were often better fed and cared for in the good homes than in many homes with a high income today and there was more discipline and less waste. "Waste not want not" was the motto of most homes. When I did my first inspection of private slaughter-houses in Britsol forty years ago I was amazed to see dozens of calves' heads for disposal in dustbins although they could be bought for 6d. or 9d. there was no demand so I called the local press boys to see me and gave them a brief talk on the value of a calf's head as a food. Within a month you could not get a calf's head in Bristol for less than 2/6!

Of course the small-holding—the family farm—was a tremendous blessing. Everyone took a hand and there was plenty to do to look after the milking cow, the calf, the pig and the chickens. Usually father worked elsewhere—in the quarry or at a nearby farm, full or part-time and financially the family was comfortable and well-fed. These small farms produced far more per acre than a big farm, and after all isn't that what matters in this little island? Talk of "economic units" in farming in mountainous Wales is just rubbish, but what do you expect when government is in the hands of economists and academics without practical experience or knowledge of human nature? Besides, plenty of physical activity keeps the body fit. It is mental worry that destroys health and happiness. An old professor friend of mine used to say that "work" was something that you did to make money so that you could later do what you liked to do. I wish he had had my experience of general practice in these parts—he would have changed his tune and I told him so.

The age of "oppressive landlordism" was passing although those who remained were still far from being "in touch" with their tenants. Since then, of course, many big estates have been dispersed but just before my time, amongst the elderly landlords, there was a practice of turning families out of their farms for not supporting the gentry in the elections. Fools ! Even today politicians all over the world think they can compel people to think their way against their own will and judgement. By laws and other means they can go so far but there is a limit. Let politicians take heed. The leaders of the chapels of Wales thought they could compel the young to conform to their own narrow standards and, as a result, the chapels are empty today. No, the attraction of the carrot is still the best way to get the donkey to win the race !

Of course a higher standard of living has brought greater happiness to many homes, but there is much to be done still for older members in their proud solitude and poverty. I am reminded of the old lady coming out of the post office, being greeted by the parson. "Good morning Mary Jones, You are out early." "Yes parson, fetching my " Lloyd George " (as the old age pension was known.) "Tut tut, Mary Jones, you talk of that man as if he had built you a railway to heaven." "I don't know about that parson but he has made the waiting room a good deal more comfortable."

I remember the old solicitor I have mentioned before telling me that a wealthy old bachelor landowner, to whom he had written months previously without getting a reply, had called to see him. The lawyer wanted the landlord to build a bath-room in a farmhouse for a widow and her large family. The landlord said "What do I get out of it ?" This got under the skin of the lawyer who jumped up and said, "Sir, this family for a hundred years has paid you for this farm over and over again. That old wooden overcoat you will be wearing one of these days won't have any pockets !" The widow got her bath-room.

Fate sometimes plays strange tricks as it did with us. I went to see an English lady, seven miles away who, whenever she came down to that part of the country, called on me to give her a check-up. When

I called on this occasion she said she was sorry that I was leaving the practice. This gave me quite a shock and I told her so because it had never crossed our minds to leave as we had two children, a lovely home, and had bought another small practice in an adjacent village and had a very good assistant with a veiw to partnership. Within a month of this incident, however, I saw an advertisement in the *Medical Journal* for a Chief Assistant M.O.H. in Bristol. After serious discussion with my wife, I was allowed to apply and within three months of the lady's prophesy I was away but I don't know whether she ever believed my denial.

Although country practice was a serious business it also had its humorous side. On one occasion I was summoned to attend a maternity case the best part of a mile up a mountainside. There was no hope of getting a car to the place but, at the bottom of the hill, grazing amongst the gorse was a donkey. I caught it and rode up along the foothpath in style. By the time I reached the top, bush-telephone had operated and a small party, including all the family, except the patient in labour, were at the front door to greet me.

On another occasion I was called to see an old lady who had been seriously ill with asthma for several days and was quite exhausted. I was prepared for drastic treatment and I took a bottle of chloroform and a piece of lint and put her under the anaesthetic. When the spasm was over I waited for her to recover. She was free from an attack for many weeks. I came across this treatment by pure chance. In 1919 I was summoned, when a medical officer in the R.A.F., to attend one of the officers who was billeted eight miles from the air station. It was about 2 a.m. I picked up my bag and jumped into a service car and when I entered the bedroom I found my patient suffering from a bad attack of asthma of several days duration. I opened my bag and, alas, it was the 'other bag' containing splints and anaesthetics. Now my experience as a resident anaesthetist at the Middlesex hospital gave me enough knolwedge and experience to realise that I could do nothing but good if I anaesthetised him. This I proceeded to do and when the spasm had subsided I watched till he had recovered from the effect of the chloroform. He was free from attacks for several months. I thought I had discovered a simple remedy for long, severe attacks of asthma but when later I consulted my bible (*Osler's Principles and Practice of Medicine*) there it was—recommended as the correct treatment under such circumstances.

One evening we received two calls within minutes of each other for two maternity cases. My wife went to one and I to the other. We went in the same direction, in the same valley about a mile apart but each some distance up the hillside on opposite sides of the valley. In the early hours of the morning after watching the slow progress of my case for a couple of hours I decided to take a walk. It was a lovely moonlight night and I thought I would see how my wife was getting on with her case. Half a mile down the lane I met my wife who had had the same idea. She came back with me and ultimately delivered both cases.

During our student days we had been warned about the difficulty of ' prognosis ' or, in simpler language, prophesying the course and result of disease. There are so many factors involved. At the same time it is most important to maintain the morale of the patient. I remember well a farmer in his sixties coming to consult me about indigestion. He had what should have been a white trimmed beard, badly stained with tobacco juice. At once I said "How do you expect not to have indigestion when you chew that stuff? That is poison and is bound to shorten your life. Stop it." "Doctor", he replied, "I came here for a bottle of medicine to ease my indigestion not to have my habits changed. I have been chewing tobacco since I was nine and I intend to continue for the rest of my life. I have had excellent health thank you, and anyway I only chew four ounces a week." I gave him a bottle. I never saw him again as a patient because we left the neighbourhood. Soon after my retirement I read in the local paper that this same man had died at the age of ninety five ! I wonder if it really had shortened his life ! Anyway a good doctor should always be a bad prophet !

CHAPTER III

BRISTOL IN PEACE AND WAR, 1928—1956

WE had been in general practice for three years and felt very satisfied with our achievements so far. The practice had grown from nothing to keeping us both busy every day and a good part of many nights but I had to confess that my health was not keeping up to it as well as I would like. Besides, we now had two children—a girl and a boy and it was no easy matter to run a house, look after a family and carry on with general practice. So my wife was not able to help as much as she would have liked and there was a further handicap of unsatisfactory staff. During our third year the doctor at the little seaside resort of Abersoch had decided to leave in search of a bigger practice. We had purchased his practice and settled a young assistant there with a view to partnership. That, had not, as we expected, reduced our load but rather increased it and this was our dilemma when I was reading the *British Medical Journal* in bed one morning—I think it was a Sunday, in the beginning of 1928. I called to my wife, "How would you like to go back to Bristol ?—they are advertising for a Chief Assistant Medical Officer of Health." There was a murmur of uncertain assent and, on the spur of the moment, I phoned up a former colleague who was the senior assistant in the school medical section and he advised me to apply. A few weeks later I was greatly surprised to find myself on the short list. The date for the interview was fixed and I arranged to take a patient to Bath to fit in with my interview. When I arrived in Bristol I thought that my chance of being appointed was not good although I had very extensive clinical and laboratory experience. The interview went off very well as I felt perfectly relaxed for I thought my hopes were slight. However, I was summoned back and offered the appointment. It took me what seemed like five minutes to answer—in those few seconds all the problems that faced me were present '*en bloc*'—another move for the family from a lovely home—to quit a life that I was enjoying as also was my wife—to find a new home in Bristol and to sacrifice my independence once again. However, I replied "I accept and thank you very much for placing so much confidence in me—I won't let you down ; I would not have applied if I had not intended to accept."

I wired my wife, "Sell the practice and be prepared to return to Bristol." So it was that we left the happy life in my native heath. My father and mother who lived near us said not a word but intense feelings are often shown by silence.

My appointment caused much annoyance to the career public health doctors. The Chief Assistant was expected to reorganise the port health service and the Ministry of Health did not consider that crossing the Channel or the ferry to Anglesey were sufficient experience. Perhaps they had not thought that a new young mind on the problem might have possibilities. They refused both recognition and to pay the grant towards the port health salary. The City Council, however, took up the challenge and told them to keep their money. Dr. Charles White on the Ministry staff, who later became Medical Officer of Health to the City and Port of London, was sent down to "inspect" me. He stayed a few days and we remained excellent friends for the rest of his life. When he returned to London my appointment was recognised by the Ministry and the port health services were reorganised. The Ministry did not hesitate to waive the need for an advertisement when approached by the City Council about my appointment as Medical Officer of Health two years later.

I was not the only one surprised by my appointment as Chief Assistant but when I look back I can see that the appointing committee had in mind my varied experience for I had had years of hospital appointments in a first class London hospital. I had been engaged in laboratory and ward cancer research for three years and had also been in general practice on my own. This experience, although it could not be included for pension purposes, is essential as backbround training to the post of medical officer of Health. The other applicants had entered the public health service early without this experience and their training therefore was limited.

At the beginning of 1930, within two years of my appointment as Chief Assistant Medical Officer of Health, my chief, Dr. R. A. Askins, was approached and accepted the appointment of Chief Medical Officer to Southern Rhodesia. A considerable amount of persuasion was used to try and keep him in Bristol because he was an efficient administrator and a far-sighted Chief Medical Officer. However, it was all to no avail and one day the Town Clerk sent for me and asked if I would accept the appointment of Medical Officer of Health of Bristol if it was offered to me. Did I think I could do it ? I replied that

Dr. Askins had been away on a course for three months and I had found no difficulties, and added, "With your assistance and your confidence in me I cannot see why I should not accept." I said too, that I had already been placed on the short list for a Metropolitan London Borough. And so it was that the City Council decided to approach the Ministry of Health to waive the clause that they should advertise the appointment. In June 1930 I was appointed Principal Medical Officer in charge of the Health Department, the School Health service and Port Medical Officer for Avonmouth and Bristol. I was thirty four years of age and had no medical assistant on the Public Health side of the Department for another four months.

But first of all let me say a little about Bristol as I saw it in 1928 when I started my work as Chief Assistant. I became aware that some of the services being provided for the people had been, and were being, pioneered by voluntary agencies and, having had first-hand experience of this voluntary work, I realize now that very few people remember today how much we owe to these pioneers. Local authorities have, under the law, limited powers only, especially in regard to the expenditure of money. There was good sense, therefore, in voluntary agencies experimenting and demonstrating the possibilities and the benefit that could follow from their actions. With this "instrument" of experience in their hands they could persuade the government to give local authorities adequate powers to deal with the problem. In Bristol there was a charming lady, Miss Townsend, who helped to start most of the welfare services including the open-air schools, infant welfare centres, occupation centres for mentally handicapped children and district nursing. I was fortunate in getting to know Miss Townsend and her pioneer workers very well.

The open-air school was where delicate children could be taught and have a mid-day meal provided. For this a site was obtained by voluntary subscription and temporary buildings were erected and furnished. After a while the local education authority provided the staff but there was no money available to have more than one such school for about sixty pupils. However, the bandstands in the parks were not used during the winter and they were lent and used for open-air classes so that the benefit was there for all to see. Today, all schools should be open-air schools and the solid, old hygienic built-for-eternity so-called "schools" should have been completely replaced.

The infant welfare-centres were started in Bristol as milk centres for poor mothers and children and later were extended to include medical and nursing help for mothers. In 1928 nearly all these centres were run by the Infant Welfare Association, grants being paid by the local authority to cover some of the cost. Today most of these clinics are held in new '*ad hoc*' buildings in different parts of the city instead of church halls or other unsuitable premises.

Occupational centres were for mental defectives unfit to attend ordinary schools. There is nothing more distressing to the parents in any home, particularly if the house is small, than to have a mentally defective child about the place doing nothing. A centre was established by voluntary subscriptions and instructors, usually craftsmen or women employed to encourage and train these children in matters of hygiene and simple occupations. Today this is a statutory obligation on all local authorities.

District nursing grew into a noble service in Bristol, some thirty five strong and many of the women were Queen's nurses. Later, trained nurses and midwives were employed by the local authority to cover all areas of the City. I was President of the District Nursing Association for twenty five years until the service was taken over by the City and I hope I played a small part in bringing the services of the voluntary organisation and the local authority together.

The Midwives Act of 1936 made it obligatory for local authorities to provide an adequate service of qualified midwives in their area. At that time there were fifty-eight private midwives practising in the City and earning only a miserable wage after paying their own expenses. Those who were under retiring age could, under this act, become direct employees of the local authority. Those who were over the retiring age could either retire voluntary or be retired by the authority. If they chose the former I think they receive one year's compensation but, if they were compulsorily retired by the authority they received three years' compensation. As their average earnings were well under £80 per annum their maximum compensation would have been £240 and no pension. I interviewed all the midwives concerned and explained the conditions to them and they all agreed to be "sacked". Dr. Askins, my predecessor, often used to say that when he took office the midwives were under the supervision of the Chief Constable who was Inspector of Midwives !

In 1930 the seventy-five slaughter houses in Bristol were privately owned and were mostly unsatisfactory. I remember in one instance the animals had to be driven through the front door of the house, past the stairs, through the kitchen to a room in the back which was called "the slaughter house". These animals were regarded as quite a "good" spectacle for the children and adults in the neighbourhood. The problem was that if the City Council closed all these places they would have to prove, after a public enquiry, that they really were unfit and then they should have to pay compensation according to the value of the business. Besides, they would have to provide alternative slaughtering facilities for the butchers affected by these closures. This was ultimately undertaken by the City Council and a new abattoir provided after preliminary work and much planning by the staff of the health department. The question of stunning the animals by electric shock before slaughter has worried me a good deal over the years. If stunning is to avoid causing pain to the animal when it is killed I doubt if it attains that object. I am satisfied that bleeding would be much less painful because then the blood fails to enter the brain and consciousness is soon lost without any pain except for the skin wound.

On the other hand a person who has received a severe electric shock never wants to suffer from that experience again. Of course there is no mess with the stunning method and it is soon over, but in fact this gives greater consideration to the feelings of the people who are doing or watching the slaughtering than it does to the 'feeling' of the beast which is to be killed.

I expressed these views to the Health Committee, to show what could be said in favour of the Jewish method of slaughtering because arguments against it had been made so often. Thereafter I was approached by the Jewish community for an article in their paper on these lines. That is what comes of talking about "possibilities" and "probabilities" as if they were facts!

Before the City Council took over the hospital service from the Public Assistance Committee in 1930 there was only a limited ambulance facility available, namely a few for infectious diseases only. The Public Assistance Committee also had a few to convey urgent pauper cases but the remainder of the service was provided by voluntary organisations, mostly by St. John's ambulances who provided a cheap service as far as the ratepayers were concerned. The attendants were trained by St. John's and it was quite efficient but hardly adequate. Soon after my appointment I was approached by a trades' union official about the wages of the ambulance staff. He did not think that

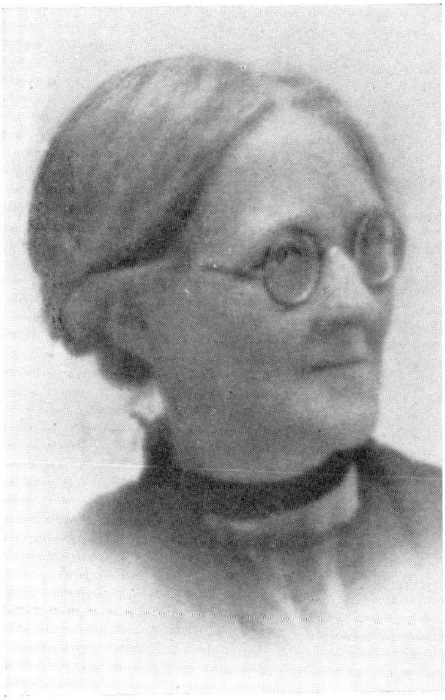

Mother in 1930

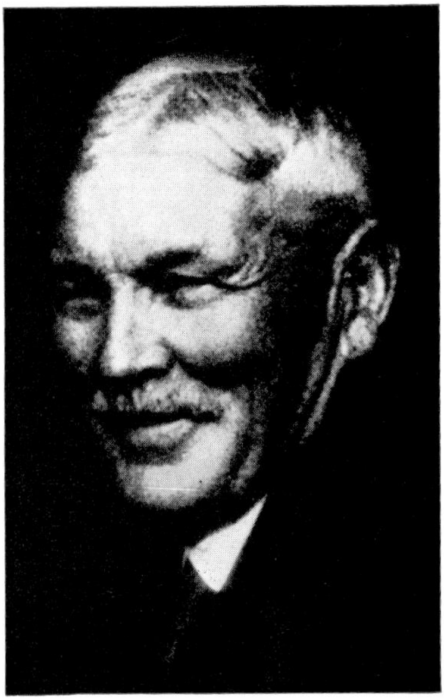

My father in 1934

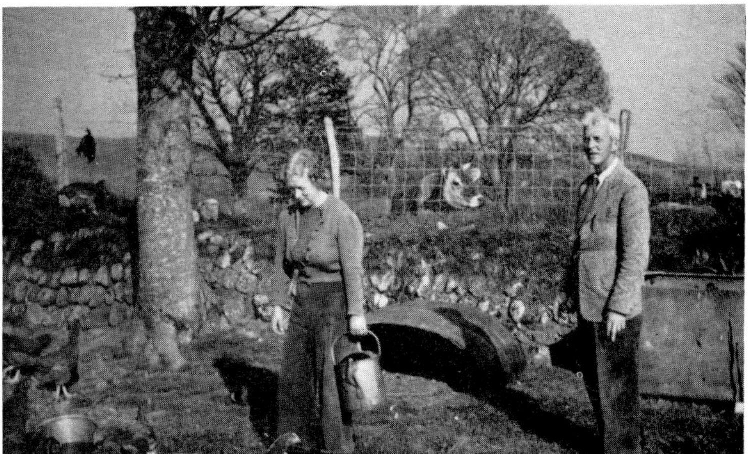

"The Farmers" under the watchful eye of one of the Jerseys

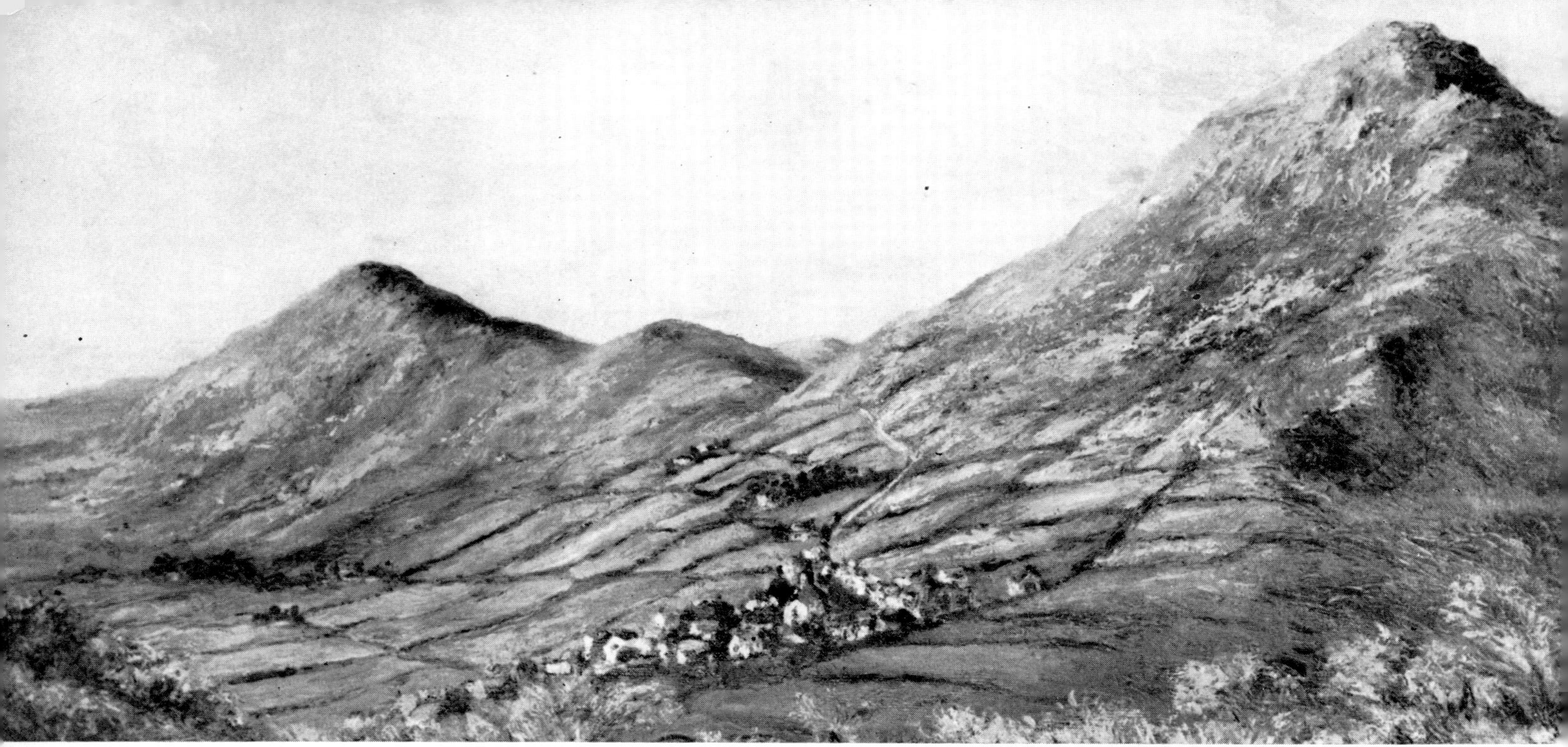

My birth place under Tre Ceiri
[*from a painting by Joan*]

22/6d. a week for the attendant and 25/- for the driver were sufficient for a family man to bring up a wife and four children. He suggested at least 2/6 a week extra for each! I sent him away with the suggestion that he should put a case for at least 30/- a week as a reasonable minimum. After receiving his reply I submitted a scheme for the Council whereby all future ambulance staff should be qualified drivers and each possess a first-aid certificate before they were appointed and I suggested a graded scheme with the minimum of 30/- but increasing with years of service. This was of great value when the ambulance service was developed as it formulated the lines on which it should progress. A few years ago I gave an address to the ambulance Service Association at their annual meeting but most of them knew nothing about the early development of their service in this country, nor do people in general appreciate the part played by voluntary organisations in pioneering this public service.

In 1928 bad housing was a terrible scourge in Bristol. There were areas where it was not safe to walk alone at night although during an outbreak of smallpox in the slum areas of the City I walked about carrying my black bag and never met any trouble. Policemen always paraded in pairs in these areas and I saw more immorality during those years both in the streets and the in homes than I have ever seen since. Why should there have been so much illegitimacy? How could it be otherwise when families slept four or five in a bed? I remember one fairly large three-storeyed house with fourteen rooms inhabited by fourteen families—about sixty human beings—a house condemned as unfit for human habitation, bought by a syndicate for a song and bringing in an income of over ten pounds a week. I was convinced that a healthy family could only be developed if it had a healthy home.

The present generation knows nothing of the dangers and damages to health that existed in those days only forty years ago. There were nearly 1,500 cases of diphtheria with about one death a week in Bristol alone—a dreadful disease for any doctor to treat, yet many doctors today have never seen a case. Over 700 cases of tuberculosis were notified in one year with 450 deaths among several thousands on the register. Six out of every ten babies born died before reaching the end of their first year. It now gives me great pleasure to compare these figures with those for 1955 when I retired by which time fewer than two out of every hundred babies died under one year of age.

As a result of immunisation which had been started in 1930, no case of diphtheria had occurred for six years and there were fewer than four hundred cases of tuberculosis and only sixty deaths. The vast improvement in health that these figures show must have meant a corresponding increase in happiness in the homes and this, after all, is the main aim of a health service.

I wonder how many young people today have experienced unpleasant contact with bugs and fleas in their homes? They were often found in old houses in Bristol in the early days of my stay in the City. The chief sanitary officer used to describe to the health committee and Press in vivid and dramatic terms how these bugs dropped from the ceilings at night onto the occupants of the rooms. A real breakthrough in getting rid of this menace came towards the end of the war when Lethane was used. Sawdust was soaked with this chemical and laid on the floor of these infested houses and the rooms shut up for forty-eight hours. This usually did the trick and was much safer than fumigation but later on D.D.T. replaced Lethane because it was much more convenient to apply. Many of these old houses were demolished under the slum-clearance schemes.

As a result of revolutionary changes in local government following the Act of 1929 it became apparent that a laboratory service was required to meet the needs of the public health in the city as well as in the city hospitals. My research and laboratory experience at the Middlesex Hospital satisfied the University authorities that a Preventive Medicine department could be established under the Medical Officer of Health as Professor to include all bacteriology for the University teaching and research purposes as well as the public health side. So it was decided by the City Council and the University authority jointly to appoint me as Professor of Preventive Medicine in administrative charge of all these services. In order to bring the public health field-work still closer the public analyst was included in the department. The Professor of Pathology, Dr. Walker Hall, resigned his Chair and became the first Director of the laboratory in my department of Preventive Medicine. I have a very happy recollection of working with him for he was a delightful companion with a keen sense of humour. He and his wife were very musical and would go any distance to hear Richard Tauber who, happily, lived in Bath at that time. They had a charming garden and house on the outskirts of the city and enjoyed their country life. He was followed by Dr. Alan

Gray and then by Dr. Cooper who later became Professor of Bacteriology. The hospital laboratory service was developed by allocating staff from the department to be responsible for the routine work in the subsidiary laboratories at the various hospitals. This was a most happy arrangement because it brought the staff together when they so wished in the central laboratory. They were all appointed and paid by the University which was reimbursed by the City.

In the hospitals themselves there were extensive changes. Ham Green, the infectious disease hospital, had several square wards because these held the greatest number of beds at the least capital cost ! But as Dr. Peters, the Medical Superintendent, and I pointed out, we were more concerned with the many varieties of disease and with observation cases that needed isolation. At last we prevailed upon "the powers that be" in London and we built two model units of single and double-bedded rooms, in the form of a cross with a central observation room from which all rooms could be seen and recognised according to the colour of the walls. The colour of the equipment was the same as the walls so as to limit as far as possible the spread of infection. At the same time I could not see why a smallpox unit could not be built in the same curtilage. This was a revolutionary idea but it was established, the unit being somewhat separated from the other units.

In Southmead Hospital which had been the old Poor Law Hospital it was necessary to draw out a development plan, and for this purpose Mr. Lawrence, a distinguished Bristol architect, was appointed to assist me. There were about thirty acres of land available so we had plenty of scope. The first stage was a maternity unit of a hundred beds, instead of the existing small unit for unmarried mothers. I felt sure that single and double-bedded wards would be most popular with four-bedded wards at the end of the corridor when the cases required less nursing. The buildings were to be single-storied. Professor Drew Smythe, the professor of Obstetrics, gave me every possible assistance and I appealed personally to Sir Kingsley Wood, the Minister of Health at that time, to allow the hundred bed unit to be so constructed. It was so successful that soon the University asked the City Council if it might be used as the Midwifery section of the Medical School. When the hospital was transferred to the Regional Hospital Board in 1948 approximately 3,000 babies were born in the unit annually. The next necessity was a modern building for a nurses' home and the first section was built at a new entrance to the west of the hospital.

When Southmead hospital was appropriated in 1930 I approached the Professors of Clinical medicine, Surgery and Obstetrics to ask if the University would form an advisory committee to help me plan the future development and as there was ample land available I thought that one day it might become the University hospital. But I knew too well, alas, that this was a very remote possibility for had not the Royal Infirmary and the General Hospital insisted on continuing their "tribal warfare" rather than come together and build a new hospital with a blank cheque offered by Harry Wills, the millionaire tobacco magnate ! However, ultimately each of the three professors was persuaded to be responsible for his speciality by providing the required service with his University teaching staff and they received appropriate salaries from the City Council.

My predecessor, Dr. Askins, had conceived the idea of a Central Clinic to provide a central workshop for the staff of the health department. I was thrilled with this idea and it was left to me to find a site and with Mr. Denning, the achitect, to plan the building. When the plan was complete it had to be seen and "vetted" by the Ministries of Health and Education. When the architect, the Town Clerk and I went to Whitehall with our plans we appeared before a formidable array of sectional chiefs of the departments, of Health and Education, maternal and child welfare, school health service, venereal disease, tuberculosis, a central dispensary, an X-ray service and others. Sitting next to the Chairman I was amazed to find that all the section chiefs were most determined to have separate units of their own. They argued that it was not possible to have expectant mothers being hustled about by school children, though some might be their own, and that men and women tuberculous patients should have separate entrances and so on. Ultimately I was content to leave it to the architect to plan the exits and entrances for each section. When this part of the meeting was over I told them something like this :—"When this is built I shall be operating the 'circus' and I shall lock all the entrances and exits except the front door through which all patients will enter and at a counter they will be directed to their particular unit." That is how it operates to this day.

I do not intend to follow the steps by which most of these problems were solved. I was fortunate in having two excellent chairmen,

Alderman Herbert Maggs and Alderman John Milton, who did all in their power to assist me in my plans for the six or seven years from the time I started my duties as medical officer of health. With their help and that of a progressive City Council, Bristol was put in the forefront of British Health services.

In 1938 Mr. Winston Churchill came to Bristol to speak at the Colston Hall. He was then in the wilderness for mentioning Germany as a possible enemy and Russia as being "as like her as the North to the South Pole". It was a very unpopular subject with the authorities but the hall was packed. I was fully persuaded that he was right. How often have we read in the papers or listened to the radio about matters put before us in a biassed way ! A reasonable person can recognise it as propaganda. Did not somebody say that you can deceive some of the people some of the time but you can never deceive all the people all the time ! But let these privileged authorities beware ! This world is full of ordinary people like myself who will listen to reason and are not to be fooled by half or less than half the truth.

War-time Bristol was not a pleasant place in which to live. Public Health activities had to be limited to essential services and development was out of the question. However, there was plenty of scope for new activities. I had to organise and supervise the administration of the casualty services, including the training of personnel in first aid and somewhere near forty thousand were so trained. Then there was the emergency ambulance service and the municipal hospitals with accommodation for nearly two thousand patients. Perhaps one of the busiest branches during the raids was the mortuary service where specially trained staff were employed to wash the bodies and identify them wherever possible after air raids on the city. A reserve of five hundred cardboard coffins was kept ready and nearly all the bodies were identified. These coffins also came in useful when Bath was raided.

During the late summer of 1939 I was approached by the Professor of Surgical Pathology of the Royal College of Surgeons and Lionel Whitby, Bacteriologist at the Middlesex Hospital, to see if I could help them to find headquarters for the Army Blood Transfusion Service. At that time the West Country was considered relatively safe from air attack and indeed arrangements had been made to evacuate government departments from London to Bristol. Lionel Whitby had lost a leg in Gallipoli and under Gordon Taylor had had a blood transfusion in those early days of the First World War when such treatment was in its infancy. He had returned from the war and came to the Middlesex Hospital from Cambridge to carry on with his medical studies. At that time I was Casualty Officer and for three months students received their first practical experience under my supervision at the casualty deparmtent. It was therefore quite natural that he should contact me in Bristol on being requested to organise the service. It was arranged that he should have the old maternity unit at Southmead Hospital, which had by this time been replaced by the new hundred bed unit on condition that he also organised a civilian blood transfusion service for Bristol and district. This is still in operation to the present day. That is the true version of the West Country Blood Transfusion Centre at Southmead Hospital from a war time emergency.

Professor Hey Groves and myself explained the scheme on the radio and were the first to appeal on the radio for donors. My wife joined the service and served as Captain in the R.A.M.C. for four years. It is estimated that in that time she took some 50,000 pints of blood for use for civilian and army requirements.

A memorable evening at the Colston Hall was when Group Captain Guy Gibson of the R.A.F. was present. I well remember having a long chat with him about the famous "dam-busting" raid when he was there at the Hall appealing for blood donors for the Army Blood Transfusion Corps. He had had as much flying as he wanted and intended taking up politics. How many of those delightful, courageous young men did we lose. We would do well to ponder how much the nation had suffered as the result of their loss.

Perhaps the most miserable day of our lives was the day when my wife and I took our four children to the ship at Liverpool when they were being evacuated to Canada. This was in 1940 when our cities were being bombed by the Germans and Bristol was one of their targets. We had given the matter serious consideration and when there was a Government appeal to send as many children to the Dominions as possible and a scheme was planned to make suitable arrangements, we finally decided to let the children go to Canada, to Toronto, where the mother of a friend had offered to give them a home. It was a dreadful day—the ugliest of our lives.

However, when they did reach Canada they found a very friendly welcome and much kindness in Toronto. Each of the children was placed in a different home and in each case the foster-parents did their utmost to make them feel that they were really "at home". The children made lifelong friends and we are glad that they have been able to return the hospitality by having the chance to welcome their war-time parents and friends to their own homes in this country.

One of the most difficult problems Bristol had to face was the evacuation of several thousands of school children into the adjacent counties. Shelter life was not conducive to cleanliness and the staff of the school medical service had to see that no child was evacuated without a thorough inspection especially as regards cleanliness. Fortunately with the help of Dr. Kearns of Long Ashton Horticultural Research Station who, afterwards became its Director, this was accomplished. Dr. Kearns had come to our rescue when blitzed tins of food and other goods had been fly-infested by advising us to mist spray with Lethane 693 special. He had used it without any risk to health when spraying fruit trees. A weak solution in liquid paraffin he assured us would kill all vermin and nits in the hair. And so with a hundred or more nurses and helpers all the children evacuated were "Brilliantined" with Lethane liquid parafin before they left Bristol. The experiment was a tremendous success and we boasted that we evacuated all the children free from vermin.

Looking back, our wartime experience confirms the historic fact that when civilisation receives a setback hygiene suffers. The reverse is equally true—health education is a civilising influence as Mohammed and John Wesley fully appreciated—the latter when he distributed pamphlets in the towns on the care of health and the treatment of illness.

Attempts were made to bring cheer to blitzed Bristol by visits of people outside the city. King George and the Queen came to see us several times after the raids and on one or two occasions they narrowly missed being caught in one. Mr. Winston Churchill was Chancellor of the University and also paid several visits. On one occasion he was coming to attend a Degree Ceremony and it was a strange coincidence that the Great Hall of the University where the ceremony was to be held should have been bombed and set on fire the night before. However, that did not deter him nor would he hear of the ceremony taking place elsewhere than in the smoking ruins. Maybe his speech after granting the degrees was the worst I ever heard him make. He stamped and grunted across the platform and I could not remember anything he had said but we could all see and sense what he felt.

Among our many visitors was a young Canadian sailor who had just escaped after being torpedoed. A raid came the evening of his arrival and we sheltered in our air raid shelter in the garden. He made no secret of the fact that he much preferred the experience to being torpedoed.

Two Canadian fighter pilots of the Battle of Britain were trying to reach us when they were caught in a raid and found beds in a small hotel near the station but they cut short their stay, preferring to be on duty fighting in the air !

Bishop Woodward whose home had been bombed and whose precious library had been destroyed was having a meal with us one evening. When he arrived I had to tell him that I had had the "pre-warning" which came to a few of us when the "beam" was on Bristol for the pathfinder German bomber. But on that occasion we had very little time before the raid started. We had a hurried meal and he insisted on walking home in case fire destroyed his few remaining books. It was a good half-mile to walk and the indenciaries were falling so I insisted he should wear one of my steel helmets. I had two for different occasions—one with C.S. printed on it and the other with M.O.H. I gave him the one with C.S. on it, the C.S. standing for Casualty Service. He wanted to know what it meant if anyone tackled him so I replied, "As far as you are concerned, Bishop, it means 'Christian Scientist'."

The kindness of several local authorities adjacent to bombed Bristol and its people has probably been forgotten by most by now but I still remember them well, especially little Sidmouth in Devon which went out of its way to try and give a holiday to a few distressed Bristolians.

Lest I become too serious and forget some of the more humourous and happy incidents during my career in Bristol here is one that I remember. It was on the occasion of the visit of Rear Admiral Gordon Taylor to Bristol during the war in 1944. One of the American armies had its headquarters in the City and I numbered among my friends many of the officers. Some of these friendships have lasted a lifetime. As a little change it was arranged that a film on chest surgery, then in a pioneering stage, should be shown at a cinema and I was asked to organise the show and to take the chair. I was delighted to find that my old chief at the Middlesex Hospital, Rear Admiral Gordon Taylor, would be talking about the film. The cinema was full of doctors, nurses, St. John's and Red Cross attendants and many first-aid workers who were interested. We expected a few casualties as a result of watching the gory scenes and indeed we got them, but the casualties were all St. John's and Red Cross attendants who were attended to by members of the audience ! That evening I arranged a little party of senior American doctors in my house to meet the Admiral who was then Vice-President of the Royal College of Surgeons. He had just returned from Russia after being commissioned by the College to present two or three honorary Fellowships of the College to distinguished Russian surgeons. He was feeling very sore about his visit as there were very few present at the ceremony whilst those present appeared to have been collected together in a hurry, as he put it, from amongst charwomen and cleaners on the premises ! He was also most interesting about the fields of surgical research that were being carried out in Russia at that time. Plastic surgery was high up on the list. He was present at the "unveiling" of the result of an operation which had been performed on a soldier whose external sex organs had been destroyed by gunshot wounds. It was arranged that a pretty nurse should be present at the unveiling ceremony and to their delight the operation was a complete success for there was "life" in the new organs.

A luncheon at the Savoy, given by the Royal College of Physicians to the Prime Minister and his Cabinet colleagues and Chiefs of Staff, was a memorable occasion. Lord Moran was our President and a limited number of Fellows of the College were invited to attend—I was one of the lucky ones. This happened to be a few weeks before "D-Day". One of the first people I saw was Air Chief Marshall Tedder. He had been my commanding officer at Bircham Newton air station in 1919 and I had the responsibility and pleasure of looking after Mrs. Tedder and her two children. This was the first occasion that we had met since then. I invited him to spend a day or more with us to rest—"free from 'shop'." When I reached home I wrote to him to confirm the invitation and to congratulate him on his achievements which I had watched with interest over the years—he was now Deputy Supreme Commander—and to sympathise with him on the death of his wife and son Dick, both killed in plane crashes, and to wish him luck. I have a charming letter in my possession that I treasure very much asking if he might postpone his visit for the time being. It had been censored at least five times. A few days later the Allied forces invaded Europe.

I next met Lord Tedder at the New Weston Hotel in New York and we had breakfast together with Lady Tedder, his second wife, and we arranged to meet in London. One day I telephoned to him at the B.B.C. of which he was then Vice-Chairman and he called for me and took me to the Atheneum for a cup of tea. There we met many old friends, including Lionel Whitby, Master of Downing College, Cambridge and an old friend of Middlesex days. He took me across to Lord Tedder to introduce me as one who had taught him in his student days, but Tedder soon put him right by saying that he had taught me the only bit if discipline I ever knew ! The last time we met was at Cambridge during an Honorary Degree ceremony for Pundit Nehru, Lord Franks and others. I was invited because my brother was also to receive an honorary degree. The Vice Chancellor was Sir Lionel Wihtby and the Chancellor who was conferring the degrees was Lord Tedder. We had a long chat and went over old times at a reception and luncheon at Downing College after the ceremony.

When the hospitals were taken over by the Regional Board many of the ablest members of my staff also went. It had to happen in the interest of the hospitals but the organisation and camaraderie of the health department suffered. However, there was plenty to do to develop clinics and get them running smoothly, the ambulance service had to be reorganised and developed and there were housing and health education schemes to be prepared for the future in the hope that one day they would come to fruition.

With the appropriation of the hospitals the Preventive Medicine department of the University which provided the laboratory services had to be reorganised and the staff of clinical pathologists went with their hospitals. This they were loath to do but they had no option. Public health bacteriology was centralised under direct control from London but the staff had been so long in the department that it made no difference to their co-operation in routine matters and our happy relationship continued.

I was very sceptic about many of these changes but we could not stand out against them just because our own services had worked in Bristol. I hate standardisation whereby we must do it this way here, whether it works or not, because that is how it is done there, two hundred miles away. Maybe one day a little more local option will obtain !

I had always been anxious to see health centres developed where local health services and general practitioners could come together and an opportunity presented itself in a large housing-estate without a resident doctor. After the war such a centre was built to meet the needs of four or five doctors who were practising in the area. It was the first in the country and called after a famous Bristol practitioner, William Budd, who in the days before germs were discovered assumed their existence and acted accordingly. Through his efforts great strides were made in the diagnosis and treatment and more especially the prevention of typhoid fever, but like all pioneers he came up against much opposition and obstruction. However, truth will out and today we know who was right. Dr. David Davies, the M.O.H. at the time had great confidence in his views and the health of Bristol benefitted much as a result.

The health centre is on a municipal housing-estate and had a great opportunity to provide consultative and expert service to the group of practitioners working in the centre. But this idea was not approved as a principle by the hospital section of the Ministry of Health or the Hospital specialists. They insisted that such services must be provided from the hospitals, which were already overloaded. Lord Beveridge came down to Bristol and I had his wholehearted support to try and obtain help for the practitioners in particular for diagnosis by providing X-ray laboratory services and maybe visits from specialists to health centres. The more we argued the more we were accused of being 'emotional'. No doubt a new generation will see the matter more clearly.

During the post-war period I was again fortunate in having a forward-looking and friendly chairman of the Health Committee, the Reverend Mervyn Stockwood, who did much to stimulate public opinion in the interest of public health.

CHAPTER IV

A VISIT TO AUSTRALIA, 1935

1935 was a wonderful year for my wife and me. I was invited to be the secretary of the Preventive Medicine Section of the B.M.A. at its Conference in Melbourne, Australia. Now, I had never attended a conference of the B.M.A. and I was distinctly timid at the thought of suggesting to my employers that my first experience of such should be in Australia—this was in the pre-flying days. However it occurred to me that there were more ways than one of making such a suggestion to the City and University. With the help of a delightful Town Clerk, Mr. Josiah Green, and two very loyal chairmen, Alderman Herbert Maggs of the Health Committee and Walter Bryant of the Education Committee, not only did the City Council approve of a four months leave on full pay but they also made a contribution of £100 towards my expenses. This money I put to obtaining a 16 mm. cine record of the journey which I still possess and some of which is in the official B.M.A. record of the Conference. The gift was a delicate matter. It is true that five years previously I had acted as Medical Officer of Health for six months on the salary of a Chief Assistant and later served as M.O.H. without a deputy or even a full-time Medical Assistant for nearly two years. The duties of the M.O.H. also included those of the Port Medical Officer at Bristol, Avonmouth and Portishead. The memory of public bodies, and indeed of the public generally is short, yet on this occasion there was very little opposition to my projected journey. It needed another approval, however,—from the Ministry of Health. There again a broad-minded Permanent Secretary did not stand in the way and wrote a brilliant letter which neither approved nor disapproved but left a very pleasant impression ! Sir Arthur Robinson, a brilliant mind, was always a kind and considerate friend to me in those early days when, as a very young man, I had to shoulder considerable responsibilities.

About that time, when the trip had been approved all round, the Lord Mayor telephoned me and suggested I should meet Mr. Joseph Lyons, the Prime Minister of Australia and his wife, who were coming to Bristol on a business visit. A quiet little private dinner was arranged at the Mansion House. There was no intention then that my wife should accompany me to Australia for we had four young children. However, Mrs. Lyons strongly supported the idea and persuaded my wife that evening, pointing out that she herself had left eleven children behind in Australia. And so arrangements were made for the care of the family and for accommodation for two of us on the tour. It was a well-organised tour with about forty of us going in the Cunarder *Georgic* to New York and a smaller number through Canada to meet us in San Francisco.

On a first visit to New York, the Statue of Liberty and the skyscrapers are always most impressive. Although I have made this journey several times since, a thrill of excitement takes hold of me every time the ship approaches the outer circle of New York. Had not my grandparents with their family of six daughters and one son, arrived in New York two years before I was born ? I wonder what it looked like in those days. There certainly were no skyscrapers then.

Elsewhere my wife and I have written a full unpublished diary of this round-the-world tour and it would take too long to tell of it here. Yet there are several interesting and amusing incidents which I cannot ignore in this account such as the police escort in New York with the sirens and the traffic making way. This sort of thing cannot happen in Britain except when Kings, Queens or Presidents and such are being entertained.

After New York, Chicago was a name with which to conjure. I cannot quite recollect what I expected before my first visit because it was the "City of Gangsters." As a child I had heard of a tinned-meat magnate who had disposed of his wife by pushing her into the 'process'. Would I look suspiciously at every passer-by and say, *sotto voce*, "there goes a gangster !" I remember my first visit to London with my country-born and bred father and pointing out to him a notice in the lift "Beware of pickpockets" ! He said quietly to me in Welsh, "You point one out to me trying his antics and I'll give him something to think about." I have visited Chicago several times since and have very happy memories of enjoyable times and good companionship. To some of these occasions I will refer again later on, but there are two particular incidents which stand out. One was our visit to the stockyards where we saw mass-production and specialization of employment that I had never contemplated in my wildest dreams. There was a man in a small pen passing a pig through a hole to the next pen at the rate of one a minute, if I remember rightly. The man in the next pen passed a ring attached to a chain round the left hind leg of the pig and swung it on the big wheel—one a minute. At the other end of the big wheel was another man who steadied the beast for the man next to him to stick and bleed it. And so the process went on until at the other end of this huge industry were pretty girls in pretty uniforms packing up smoked and unsmoked bacon. We had a very tasty tender steak for lunch !

The other incident was when my wife and I, by arrangement, met five pretty girl cousins of mine on the steps of Marshal Field Museum on the Boulevard Michigan. "And why, Bob," they said after each had been soundly kissed, "have you not been to see us before ?" "But you have only just put away Al Capone and I did not think it was too safe !" "Oh, but what about babies in cardboard boxes at Brighton—this country is much more civilised!" Such is the news that keeps countries of the world "closely informed", on how the ordinary people live ! Alas. My wife was very firm in her denial when I thought I recognised another girl cousin dancing in a cabaret show at the Stevens Hotel later. And I was so sure she gave me a smile of recognition !

Albuquerque—a strange name for a desert city. It was said to be built around a sanatorium in the days when tuberculosis was a scourge. It was a delightful city surrounded by mountains from which it obtained its ample water supply which it badly required. As far as I can remember, like most other cities in summer in the southern U.S.A., sprinklers were essential for anything like a grassy lawn to be maintained. Let us never complain about our ample rain !

As we were entering our hotel in Albuquerque, a shortish dark-haired middle-aged man came up to me and said "Are you English ?" "No," I said, "I'm Welsh." Great was his astonishment. So I asked him, in Welsh, "are you Welsh ? Where do you come from ?" "Yes," he replied, "I come from Caernarvonshire." "So do I". "Are there many Welsh people with you ?" "About half a dozen, I should say. Here comes a Welsh lady from Liverpool". Half an hour later they were still talking—they had been attending the same Sunday School in Liverpool more than twenty-five years before. An engineer by profession, he had only come to Albuquerque for the day to visit his daughter. The last I saw of him on this occasion, was chasing after the train and waving his handkerchief and his eyes looked very wet to me. Eight years later, in 1943 whilst on tour with the party from the

American Public Health Association, I was billed to speak at Albuquerque. We went straight from the train to the hotel to meet the reception committee. In the vestibule, a short dark elderly man pushed his way through and asked "Can I speak to Dr. Parry ?" "Yes, here I am." "You wouldn't remember me." "Indeed I do. Mr. Jones from Dolwyddelen in Caernarvonshire." "What a memory," he exclaimed ; but how could I forget ! He had retired then and was living at Albuquerque but there was a suggestion that half his heart was elsewhere.

I remember Sir Mortimer Wheeler being interviewed on the radio. He came from Bradford and spoke of the city as if it were the most wonderful place in the world. "But you have retired to live in the South of England—why not in Bradford ?" "Ah" said he, "it is a wonderful place to think about but not to live in !" I suppose that is why everyone is most patriotic when he is away from his own country. But beware of disillusion if you should ever revisit old haunts after long absence ! I shall never forget one of the great mistakes of my life when I returned to my old home—where I had been born and of which I had such happy memories—to present, to the local chapel, a large self-portrait in oils of my great-grandfather, the founder of the chapel. My wife had never been to my old home and I had not revisited since leaving it more than fifty years before. We found a desolate semi-deserted old house with none of the furniture that I remembered and certainly not in the spick and span state I treasured in my memory. The old water wheel was silent and many of the trees were down. It was a sad experience indeed.

I do not wish to describe the journey from Albuquerque to San Francisco because it would take too long. We saw the Grand Canyon, one of the great wonders of nature ; and we passed through the fruit country of Los Angeles and, after a short stay and a visit to the Paramount Picture Studio, travelled on by the coast route to San Francisco. It was a never-to-be-forgotten train journey and our private little compartment was comfortable and most pleasant.

I must here say a word about the hospitality of the Americans to their guests—and not only if they are V.I.P's. There are no more generous people in the world than these people in their own country—that is certainly my experience after several visits and fairly long sojourns in the country. When we arrived in San Francisco on this tour, the chairman of the hospitality committee was the Health

Commissioner, Dr. Geiger. He met the train and called for me, as the representative of the public health service in the party. In the department car with a police escort, sirens and motor cycles and all, we were rushed into the hotel and booked in. Then through China town to Dr. Geiger's house where I had my first experience of a mint julep. The incident is so vivid that I must give a detailed account of it. With me were my wife and my aunt who had been smuggled into our train compartment at Los Angeles as she was going to Berkeley to visit some friends. When we arrived at his house, he asked, "Would you like a mint julep ?" "Why not ?" Dr. Geiger and I retired to the "kitchen"—more like a laboratory—took our coats off and donned white coats. The mint julep consisted of crushed mint, a couple of slices of pineapple, ice and topping the tumbler with scotch. A very tasty and, believe me, a potent drink. "What about another ?" My caution was overwhelmed for I knew that I would be taken back to my hotel and would not have to drive myself. I left the last of my drink until we were nearly ready to leave. The journey back meant only a few minutes in the car and a short lift-ride to our hotel room. I remember taking my shoes and coat off and lying on the bed and there I found myself in the morning fresh and fit and without thirst or a headache. Some years later during the war I was travelling to London with two American officers, one from California and the other from Texas. I described this wonderful 'refresher' and almost started a civil war ! Apparently there is no national standard for mint juleps and each argued that theirs was the more potent or palatable !

Besides our reception in San Francisco by the Health Commissioner with a police escort which I have described, three little incidents stand out in my memory on that occasion. The department car in which we travelled was equipped with radio and whilst we were travelling the Health Commissioner received information of eleven cases of antimony poisoning, which had just been transferred to hospital, with full details. When I made a point of dwelling on this in my talk to the City Council on my return and stressed the future value of radio, most of my audience smiled and afterwards referred to it as another new-fangled American idea. This was thirty-four years ago.

As we were preparing to leave the hotel at San Francisco to board the ship, *s.s. Aorange*, my mother's only brother, Morris, his wife and his son came over to see us. They had driven down some 300—400 miles from a town called Tranquility in California. In 1949 when I

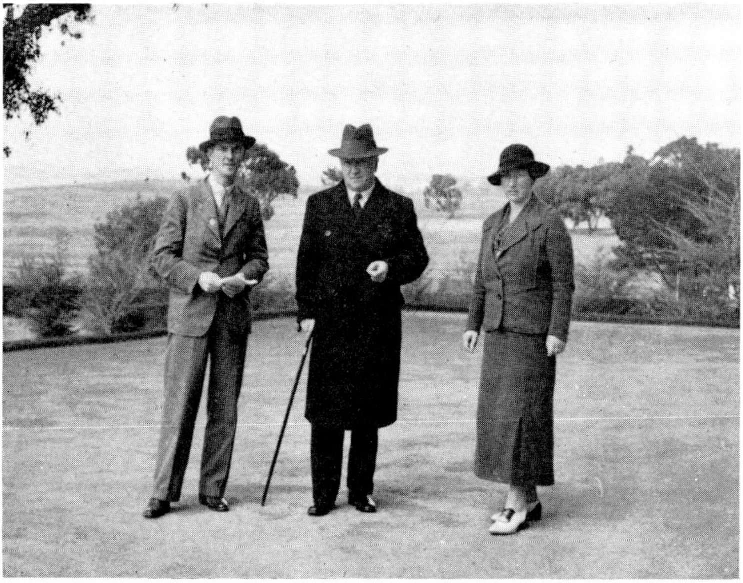

With Mr. Joseph Lyons, the Prime Minister, in Canberra, 1935

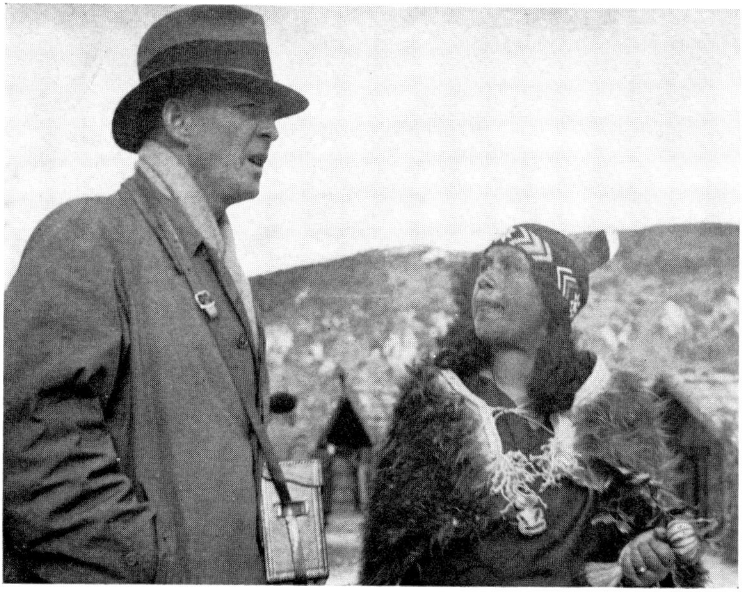

Talking to a Maori lady in Rotorua (1935)

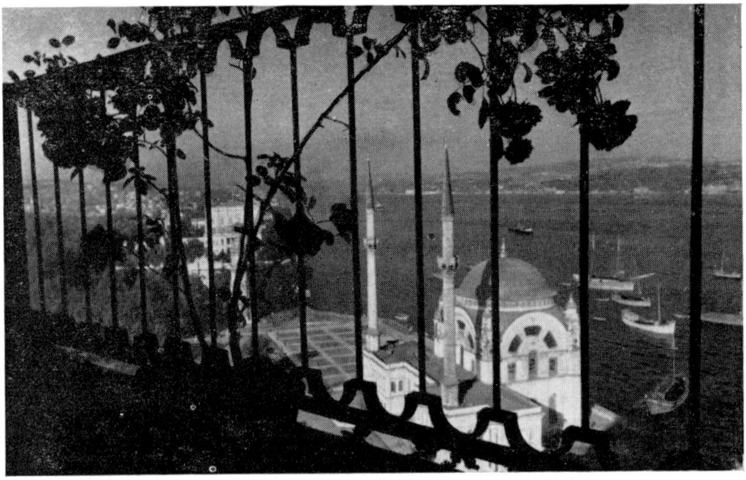

A view of the Bosphorous from friend's garden

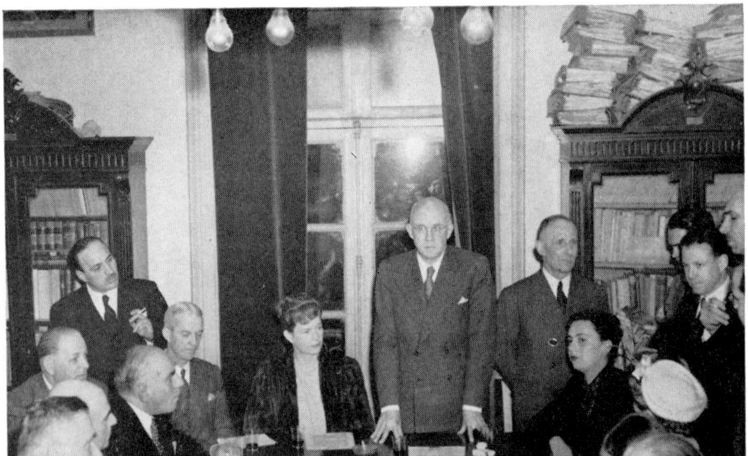

Oscar Powell addressing a meeting of doctors and others
in Athens

was with the American Mission to Greece a young American administrator was working in the same office. He came from California. I told him of a place I felt sure he had never heard of—Tranquility ! He came from that town and knew my uncle and his family ! I was speaking in San Francisco eight years later in 1943, and I again saw my uncle and his son but my aunt was dead. He also spoke a good deal about the old home,—to which I have already referred. I am glad he cannot see it now—or can he ?

The third incident was when a Welshman brought to the ship a basket of the most wonderful fruit I have ever seen to wish us well on our journey. He was the British Consul and a distant cousin. It was a great surprise as I did not know he was in that part of the world.

Maybe it was Honolulu in the Hawaian Islands that impressed us most of all. The climate was perfect—sunny without being too hot—with the wide expanse of sand and the substantial waves that came bounding towards the shore with numerous little rafts and boards all with human figures standing or lying on them. The ship was met well outside the harbour by large numbers of young Hawaian boys seen clearly from the decks swimming at different depths as well as on the surface of the crystal clear water. The passengers on the ship dropped coins into the water and the young lads dived after them and often caught them in their mouths. There was no limit to our admiration of their feats and we demonstrated loudly. The ship was greeted on shore by a band playing Hawaian guitar music and a party of the local inhabitants came on-board carrying garlands of flowers which they proceeded to slip round the necks of their visitors. My wife and I were doubly welcomed in this way for the Health Commissioner brought a couple to cheer us in when we landed.

We must, of course, first of all have a go on the surf boats. Although I was not a swimmer I had complete confidence in my guide. It was just as well that I did for on our way out I was knocked clean over by a board coming on top of a wave. I don't seem to have been in the least perturbed—I remembered to stop breathing as I went down and down towards the bottom of the Pacific. Presently my guide was with me and, firstly by the leg, later by the top part of the body, he hauled me up to the surface which was not in the least unpleasant and quite an experience ! Our punishment came a couple of days later when all the skin over the exposed part of our bodies peeled off, leaving us very sore and exempting us from being "baptised" by

Father Neptune when he came aboard at the equator as we "crossed the line". Honolulu will always remain a happy memory with both of us. We heard of a Scottish couple who had come there for their honeymoon seventeen years before, and they were still there. Trust the Scots! With a couple of friends we visited a Hawaiian village and the pretty young Hawaiian lady did her best to show me how to dance the hula hula. I was not very sucecssful because I did not seem to possess a rotund middle which is a great help when you want to wobble it about. In despair the young lady placed her hand where the tummy ought to be, to try and help. Laughing of course did not help· It all appears on the 16 mm. film and is also part of the official B.M.A. film. Perhaps I should explain that my wife took the pictures!

The scenery was magnificent and quite beyond my powers of description. I remember a concert of Hawaiian music and a dinner we had at the Hawaiian Hotel that evening where we also became acquainted for the first time with an avocado pear which we did not appreciate at the time but learned to enjoy later.

When we arrived at Fiji it was raining and they seemed to have been expecting it, for everyone carried an umbrella! The native Fijians, with their fine crops of dark hair, their big, tanned bodies and their bare feet were objects of admiration to us. One such, a sergeant of the police, paraded placidly along the quay whilst our ship was docking. The Governor had arranged a fire-walking ceremony for our benefit and a dance by the Fijian heroes. A large cup of Kava was then handed round for us to drink. I have never investigated thoroughly how this drink was prepared and felt there was hardly any need to, after surviving sampling it. Two of our party, a neurologist and a professor of anatomy were selected to examine the firewalkers before and after. The large stones in a pit which had been coveerd with burning timber for twenty four hours were certainly hot because I threw a few leaves on them and they went up in smoke. A party of half-a-dozen firewalkers deliberately walked over the stones. According to our experts there was no sign of a burn on their feet and they argued the why and wherefore all the way to Australia. The issue almost divided the party between the neurologist with a psychological explanation, and the anatomist who opted for thick skin. Some of us shook our heads and said "a bit of both maybe."

We arrived in Auckland, New Zealand, in the late afternoon. It was really a beautiful rin-in through the bay to the harbour and a reception had been arranged for us at the University. At the party after a few drinks we were challenged to go with our host in his car to the top of Mount Eden and really see Auckland and its bay at midnight. It certainly was worth seeing but I doubt if I would repeat the experience of being driven at midnight after a cocktail party. Rotorua with its hot geysers and its dancing Maoris is certainly worth seeing and is indeed a sight which could never be forgotten. A hot-water stream running within a few feet of a cold one permitted the villagers to do their washing in hot water and rinse in the cold by merely turning round in their seats. Saucepans with potatoes to cook and kettles to boil were to be seen about ; but best of all was the sight of a fisherman hooking a trout and, whilst it was still on the hook, swinging it into a hot stream to cook ! Not so pleasant was the bubbling, boiling, black mud and I should be very loth to have to care for small children in such a place. Certainly one of the wonders of the world and what economy in fuel !

From Auckland in New Zealand we went on to Sidney in Australia and when we arrived there we decided not to proceed direct to Melbourne but to join a small party and take a service-car to see the Blue Mountains. And what a ride ! It is difficult in a quick run to take in the beauty of the scenery but it is impossible to forget the view from the top of the spiral drive, past the blue lake to the Guest House. Certain incidents left an indelible impression on our memories and that drive was certainly one of them. The facilities offered to campers and picnickers to stop and enjoy themselves was another. How different from this country where in summer time it is almost impossible for visitors to find room to stop much less for the children to have a run.

At the Guest House near the Jenolan Caves we received every possible hospitality and kindness, even to the extent of a hot-water bottle in our beds for it was none too warm at night. We visited the magnificent Jenolan caves and heard the kookaburra, or laughing jackass, and saw a lyre bird in captivity.

As for Sydney, what a fine city it is and what a harbour ! We learned afterwards that a certain amount of jealousy existed between the different cities and the inhabitants of Melbourne said that the Sydneyites worshipped their harbour so much that they started the Lord's Prayer with "Our harbour which art in Sydney." It was well worth seeing with its wonderful bridge and its little Pinchgut island where convicts were once chained and were almost submerged when the tide came in. In the Koala Bear Park we actually saw several little bears eating away at their eucalyptus leaves. They certainly are adorable and make wonderful pets if they can be given the correct food.

Then came Melbourne where we were shown exceptional hospitality. We boarded the train at Sydney and had to change at Aldbury because the gauges of the railways were then different in New South Wales and Victoria. (They have been standardised since). We arrived in Melbourne after an all-night journey, and our memories of that city are all happy ones. We visited a big chicken farm ten miles or so out of the city which was managed by two brothers who, we were told, had been sacked from the municipal farm nearby because they could not read notes sent to them by the foreman. They at once settled down to chicken farming on the outskirts and produced about a quarter of a million chickens a year. When we went there there was a Japanese man sexing the chickens and drowning the cockerels. I remember sitting next to the Lady President of the Maternity Section of the Conference at Lincoln, Nebraska, in 1943 and when she asked me if I was interested in poultry-rearing and chicken-farms I told her I had been over the biggest in Australia in 1935. A diner opposite asked the lady how many ckickens she had reared so far that year—and this was in June—and she replied four million or so. I declared I would never again mention the "little farm" in Australia.

In Melbourne there always seemed to be great difficulty in getting taxis to and from meetings and receptions especially in the evening. Soon after our arrival we found one and after a little chat with the driver we found he had only been in Australia eight years and he came from Finsbury Park, London, which was also one of my old haunts in my student days. We had many a reminescent chat afterwards and henceforth there was always a taxi "reserved" for us which made a great deal of difference to our comfort.

One day soon after our arrival in Melbourne we received a call to the telephone at our hotel. It was an invitation from Mr. Lyons, the Prime Minister, to dinner at his hotel and a visit to the theatre with him. When we arrived in our seats the manager made a little speech of welcome to the Prime Minister on his return home and he welcomed his guests. In the interval we were taken back stage to meet the actors and actresses and it was a very pleasant evening indeed.

Before leaving I was invited to address the Sunday School at the Welsh chapel and there I found quite a strong colony of Welsh-speaking people gathered together to talk and sing.

One of the receptions was at the famous Melbourne Club. On arrival I was received with much vigour and warmth by the student President of the University Union. He had sought me out particularly because his name was Parry but I could not trace any family relationship or resemblance. He was a powerfully built young man with a crop of ginger hair and well over six feet tall. "I want to see that you are properly looked after" he said and presented me with a bottle of Scotch which he took from under his dinner jacket. I replaced it under mine but not for long for it was soon emptied with his, and his friend's assistance !

After the conference was over the Prime Minister arranged to meet us at Goulbourne and drive us to Canberra in a fast new Humber car he had brought back from England. It was a memorable run and gave us the first experience of seeing a mirage. We saw a very large lake ahead of us with a herd of cattle standing in it but we drove through this ' lake ' and there was no water. Our three days at the Prime Minister's Lodge were most enjoyable and our only regret was that Mrs. Lyons had had to return to Tasmania after their long and tiring journey abroad.

We spent very pleasant, and indeed, memorable evenings with Mr. Lyons whilst staying at the Prime Minister's Lodge in Canberra. It was a new and exciting experience to talk and listen to a ' top rank ' politician on world affairs in which he was playing a prominent part. The Italian-Abyssinian war was raging at that time in 1935 and feelings were running high between nations with there being no guarantee that the war would not spread to involve other nations. To Mr. Lyons, however, Australia was his number one treasure. He dearly loved his country and even his own career was of secondary importance. Of this I was convinced after living with him in his own home for several days. He worked hard and because of his lameness his physical activities were limited.

The future of his Government's policy towards the developing of industry in Australia was not too clear and it gave him many hours of anxious thinking. What indeed was the best policy for Australia to follow, in the interest of Australia ? Britain pressed heavily for the policy of remaining mainly agricultural to supply the needs of her small over-industrialised island. But Mr. Lyons understood the attitude of the millions of Asians who were casting envious looks at the thousands of undeveloped acres whilst they themselves were sadly overcrowded. What should his Government do? Many leading Australians were wishing very much to see millions of British people settling down in Australia and bringing with them their industries and skills and today we see that they were right. Alas that selfish interests should cloud clear vision in our own country on such a problem.

Another problem facing the Australian Government was that of broadcasting. Television had not yet arrived, but Mr. Lyons saw very clearly the great possibilities of this instrument of communication for good and for ill. To what extent should it be government-controlled or government-operated and where did private enterprise come in? Mr. Lyons was a socialist. Perhaps he had not the strong reasons for vindictive socialism which unfortunately exists in this country but when I look back I am deeply impressed with the unbiassed argument he put up on behalf of all points-of-view.

The sense of humour which Mr. Lyons possessed must have pulled him out of many a tight corner. He was excellent too at "leg pulling". His family came from the South of England and Mrs. Lyons, now Dame Enid Lyons, hailed from Devonshire—with the good Welsh name of Enid. He told amusing stories about his predecessor, Mr. W. M. Hughes, who had been the war-time Prime Minister. The easiest way to prevent the admission into the country of undesirable aliens was by the language barrier. Mr. Billy Hughes, as he was affectionately known, could always help out by asking questions in Welsh! Billy Hughes was deaf—to what extent Mr. Lyons was never quite sure—but he usually wore hearing aids and when a speech to which he had to listen went on too long he made a great show of removing the instruments and putting them on the table in front of him.

As a reminder to Mr. and Mrs. Lyons of their kindness to us and their hospitality we sent some packets of flower seeds and many years later we heard that the plants were still thriving in their garden in Tasmania.

The Prime Minister took us in his car to Sydney where we separated to go our own way. We took a service-car to see Bendigo and then travelled by the Murray River to Mildura. At Mildura on a Saturday afternoon I was taken to the Settlers Club, one of three large clubs in this new town. It was a large oblong room with a long bar counter in the middle. There must have been three to four hundred men in this "men only" preserve drinking beer as fast as they could. When the clock struck six the bell went and all drinking stopped. There was a long queue from which emerged men with their pockets full of bottles—for the weekend ! In contrast to America where attention to punctuality is not so popular the Australians were strictly punctual. No drinks were served after six o'clock except to guests and bona fide travellers. Of course, punctuality has its awkward moments—for example when we wanted to leave our hotel at Mildura to get to Adelaide the service-car left the hotel at 8 a.m. sharp and the day staff at the hotel arrived at 8 a.m. sharp. We tried to get two boiled eggs, bread and butter and tea and whilst we were eating it the service car left. We thought we were stranded but not at all. A taxi took us by a short cut to meet the service-car some six or seven miles away.

I must not forget to mention a building we saw at Wentworth said to have been built as a goal. The state Government officials could not find it because it ought to have been built at Broken Hill which is maybe one of the advantages, or disadvantages, of a large country !

Our stay in Adelaide was filled with most interesting and busy excursions to different museums, institutions and beauty spots under the guidance of D. Angus Johnson, the Health Officer and his son and of Dr. and Mrs. Southwood. Dr. Southwood was the State Health Commissioner and on one of these journeys took us to a Country Club on the Mount Lofty range overlooking Adelaide. I can still see that wonderful view of the country in the clean air ! We lunched at the Club with Sir Harry Newlands.

The time was now approaching for us to think of going home. We had sacrificed the opportunity of seeing the Orient by keeping with the party and sailing round the east coast as we were anxious to see as much as we possibly could of Australia. A train journey to Perth did not appeal for us so we sailed from Adelaide to Freemantle. We were told at the time that good sailors "went down" in the "Australian Bight" but I never was nor am a good sailor. It seems that the Indian Ocean meets the Pacific somewhere there and they try and adjust their differences. The ship was either too short or too long for it kept on the crest of the waves for two, maybe three, in succession and then down it went to the trough. It was perfectly comfortable lying flat in the bunk but then how would I watch and film the albatrosses? A quick run to deck, a snap and then down again with a glass of ginger ale waiting. I survived and managed to take several good pictures. And so to the fine port of Freemantle and sight-seeing in Perth on the Swan River. We were deeply impressed. What a wonderful country in which to live! It has everything and we seriously considered making it our home, but when a person is comfortable and happy with strong roots and family ties, cutting those ties is no easy matter. Besides, it is easier to write a book and dream about a place after a short visit than after settling down in it. It is a vast country, even now only partly explored, and one day, maybe before very long, it will be the wonder country of the world. Already flying has brought us closer together as it has the world in general. I wonder if Australians still think that when a settler goes to Sydney the first question he is asked is "How much money have you?" In Melbourne "Who are you?" In Adelaide, "What are your qualifications?" and in Perth "Come and have a drink old chap."

After our hospitable and pleasant stay in Australia we found an exciting change in our visit to Ceylon. It was unbearably hot in Colombo and that made a delightful 70 mile run by car to Kandy doubly attractive. The Buddhist priests in their gaily coloured robes, the school children, a village wedding and, most amusing of all to a health officer, a man and an elephant having bath and drink together in a river. Girls picking tea leaves—they were all sights we had never seen before but no doubt anyone could soon get used to them and then forget to mention them at all. No, it is not a question of familiarity breeding contempt but when we become accustomed to anything it is no longer "news" to the mind.

The most vivid memory I have of Aden was the smell of camels after we had been held up behind a camel train in a tunnel! There were also two other impressions—it hadn't rained for five years and they were not expecting rain for another two years. And then there was a most remarkable view of the sun setting on the sea horizon as the ship sailed out of harbour—the fiery red fierce sunset!

Then came the Red Sea without a breath of air—in an air-conditioned ship. What it must have been like in sailing days! I was not surprised to hear that many a good sailor jumped overboard never to be seen again because the heat was more than he could stand.

The run from Suez by car to Cairo, a visit to the Pyramids, tea on the Nile and the treasures of Tutankhamen were all experiences I cherish. Port Said, Malta and so to Marseilles. As we passed the Chateau d'If near Marseilles I was reminded of Pinchgut Island in Sydney narbour and Alcatraz in San Francisco Bay and thought what a state of helplessness being "installed" in any of these must be in what ever capacity. So on to Tangier, Gibraltar, Plymouth and home. When we landed at Plymouth I was interviewed by the Press.

It was raining—at the beginning of September. "What is uppermost in your mind, doctor, on arriving home from a world tour ?" "What glorious rain," was my reply, "I shall never complain about it again. We travelled through the scorched parts of southern U.S. In Australia they were complaining that thousands of animals were dying of thirst. In Aden it has not rained for five years and they were not expecting any for another two years. You know what it looks like without rain as you travel from Suez to Cairo. Yes, this rain is wonderful." It so happened that my farming father was listening to this talk on the radio in Caernarvonshire. Said he "It's all very well for him to talk like that but this is the wettest summer ever and we just cannot find a chance to get a load of dry hay in."

In 1935 Britain was at the height of her power. Wherever we went we saw British warships and the British pound was most acceptable. But we could not help feeling we were there on suffrance, because it paid them ! No one likes to see his home occupied by another. Somerset Maughan said somewhere, after his journeys through the East, that the British were respected but the French were admired. "When in course of time these peoples inevitably regain their freedom it will be interesting to see which of these emotions has borne the better fruit." We have arrived at the moment and we watch and we fear.

CHAPTER V

TOURS IN THE UNITED STATES IN WAR AND PEACE

1943 AND 1951

By 1943 we in Britain had been subjected to a severe bombardment by the Germans. There was considerable destruction evident in Bristol, referred to elsewhere, and the American armies had arrived in 1942. I first became aware of their presence when my Assistant Port Medical Officer at Avonmouth had come across three American officers on the dock-side trying to find their way about. He brought them over to my office and soon we all became fast friends. The senior officer was Colonel Howard Hutter and his record was an interesting one. He had been trained at West Point after qualifying as a Doctor and was one of the four officers sent to the Phillipines to train their army some years before the war. The senior officers of that party were Colonel MacArthur, Major Eisenhower, Major Davies, who was killed, and Major Hutter. Major Hutter married a famous dancer and film star from the Phillipines, Feli Francelli, and retired from the services to settle down in practice on Long Island. He remained the personal physician of General MacArthur when the latter retired to live in New York. His description of life in the Phillipines we found most interesting and amusing—the 100 years old Chinese egg and the "ballute" which was a delicacy—a duck's egg incubated to near full term and then hard boiled ! I shall refer to my friends the Hutters again later on.

In March 1943 I was approached by the British Information Service with a request to visit U.S.A. and talk to them about our blitzed cities. I certainly had had sufficient experience of this in Bristol. The invitation had come from the American Public Health Association and it was proposed that a party of experts should visit the different state capitals of U.S.A. where a state conference of public health workers would be in session. In this way one large central conference could be avoided. I was to be the foreign guest and I was looking forward to this very much.

Arrangements had first of all to be made for my transport so I visited the transport office of the British Information Services in

London where a large solemn man with a deep booming voice interviewed me. "How would you like to go, Doctor ?" "Well—I was in the Air Force when Alcock and Brown flew the Atlantic so I would like to go by air". "Well, this is difficult, Doctor—we only had three flying boats, one has been destroyed by the enemy, another is under repair, and the third is the other side of the Atlantic at the moment." "Why not the Queen Mary ?"

"Well, I do want to go by air. If the Americans want me to go over can't they take me ?" "That's an idea : We'll see about it."

It was to be a four-months visit so I went at once and insured my life for a substantial sum and waited. A few days later I was summoned to the American Office in London and be prepared for the journey. I was told to sit down and wait. There was no further information but later in the day I was then told to report again to-morrow.

The next day I reported back at the American Office in London with my luggage complete, ready to go via the "southern route" which I understood would be warm, and so equipped with light clothing. As the truck-full of American officers with whom I was travelling started up I realized we were heading north. The young American officer mext to me asked "Is it far ?" Remembering the poster "Don't talk" my reply was "No, quite near". We arrived at "an airport" and boarded a DC American plane fitted with bucket-seats round the cabin. Strapped in we flew fairly low and bumpily over England due north and I was violently sick as I always am on a bumpy air or sea journey. I was comforted to find myself sharing a bucket with a British Commando—although I saddened lest he and the others felt the same when the great day came for them to cross the channel !

We arrived at Pretswick and at the desk I was given my seat in an American plane to leave at 10 p.m. I boarded the plane and after we had been locked in the Captain came in and briefed us. We were flying south to Gibraltar but the enemy were shooting down unarmed planes so please don't show a light. I looked round and found I was the only civilian. Next to me sat an American Medical Colonel. I took my sleeping pills and settled down to sleep. Ten minutes later there was a bump and we had landed back at the aerodrome. The Captain came in and told us one of the engines was missing so he had turned back. We were disembarked and told that another 'plane would leave in two hours on the same route. My American medical friend was booked on it but not me. I had to wait for our 'plane to be repaired. The American friend directed me to a Nissen hut well down the air station and told me to give his name and half-a-crown a night and the room, well heated, would be mine for as long as I was stranded at Prestwick. I followed his instructions and it was so. The first night, however, seven of us were bundled into a waggon and taken to billets in the town where we were shown into a big room with six camp-beds and nothing else. I selected one in a corner and slept all night. Maybe I was not so old after all ! My companions were Norwegians and Poles. After three nights in my Nissen hut I was booked to leave at midnight and this time there was another civilian, a good deal younger than I. He later became the distinguished chairman of Yeovil Helicopter Company. The captain, the same one on the same plane, came in to brief us and said we were heading north for Iceland. He was a calm, quiet man who had spent much of his life as a tea-planter in the East. We arrived at the Reykjavik airport in the early afternoon in bright sunshine and were taken to the American officers' mess nearby. The captain told us that he could not get service for the 'plane but he hoped he could do something to get the missing engine going for it had failed again. We went round sight-seeing and then to bed. Next morning we found we had been completely snowed in by a storm during the night and it was dreadfully cold I wore all the clothing I had with me, and which was ready for Brazil ! but it depressed me to see my companions,—American commandoes and British ferry pilots, stripped and doing their daily dozen first thing in the morning. Yes, after all, I wasn't so young ! After forty-eight hours in Reykjavik we set off in sunshine once more, the missing engine still missing. I sat near the port-hole on the starboard side and after a few hours I could see the outside engine lagging and oil dripping. It was not too pleasant a sight but the rest of the view was marvellous. We hugged the coast of Greenland and could see plainly the huge mountains of ice. In no time, it seemed, we were in Goose Bay, Labrador. Snow-ploughs cleared a way for us and we had a meal but our journey was spoiled somewhat by shortage of oxygen masks and we tended to "blow up". The slow journey, with one engine missing, over lighted-up Quebec and the St. Lawrence River to Montreal, where we arrived at night, was a memorable journey. All the same I was glad to arrive safely and to find myself in the overheated but otherwise comfortable hotel. Next morning I took a plane to La Guardia airport, New York, and reported at the British Information Services in Rockefeller Centre.

This was my first experience of crossing the Atlantic by air. I cannot say it would be my choice in the future unless "the means" improved a good deal. However, I had done it and I would see what it felt like to return in the same way.

When I reported to the British Information Services in New York, I declared myself unfit for work for a week and, having heard abou my journey, they agreed. Where would I like to go ? To Canada, of course, where my four children were living as war guests. That was impossible. That was another country and the New York Information Service had nothing to do with Canada ! Well, well—I was back in Whitehall—I must shake myself free of English red tape. I reported to the Medical branch of the Rockefeller Foundation and had a warm reception. I told them my story. What part of Canada ? Toronto. When ? As soon as possible. Whilst we were still talking, Dr. Muench, whose kindness I shall never forget, came back with a return ticket by air from La Guardia to Toronto where my daughter was waiting to receive me. It was a fine tonic to see the four children and to spend a week with them—as the guest of the Rockefeller Foundation.

When I arrived back in New York I had acute frontal sinusitis. But, alas, the British Information Services nad no facilities or arrangements for medical treatment and again I had to see my friends at the Rockefeller Foundation. Next morning I received a tumultous welcome on the 14th floor of Cornell Medical Centre under Dr. Macauliffe. Forthwith to the operating theatre where Dr. Macauliffe cleared the opening to my sinus and I felt much better. I asked the pretty nurse who looked after me if they were always as cheerful and sweet to their patients. "Not really," she said, "You see, this is a women's ward usually !" I should'nt have asked, should I ?

I do not intend to describe the exciting months that followed. It was all new experience to me and came at a time when the Americans looked up to Britain. We had stood alone, we had stuck the blitz and Mr. Churchill's words were engraved on their minds. All this delivered me into their arms in a blaze of glory. In Boise, Idaho, following my after-lunch talk to a full meeting of the Kiwanis when I described very breifly a night of blitz—as a father in his own home, I was amazed to see tears and they all stood up and cheered when it was over. All very unexpected. I paid two further visits to U.S.A.—in 1951 and in 1956—and spoke at many meetings but the spell was broken.

My 1943 tour was divided into three parts—about a month to tour a few of the Eastern States and the Middle West, a month as one of a party of twelve to visit the different state capitals and then a third month as a guest of the Rockefeller Foundation to visit the different universities.

During the first part of the tour my first visit was to Hartford Connecticut and then to Bristol by car where I had a great welcome. I made my first mistake when I spoke at the Girls High School auditorium to an invited audience for about twenty minutes—it should have been forty at least. I learned later to weigh my audience better. However, they did give me the "key to the city"—a yale key with "Bristol" engraved on it. I understand they have a large works in the city where they make all kinds of keys !

Of course, my Middle West tour had to start in Chicago and there I found that most remarkable man, Dr. Herman Bundesen, the Chairman of the Board of Health and a tower of strength to me. He went out of his way to help and his generous and friendly hospitality were much appreciated. I must recount what I know about this extraordinary person, most of which I gathered from him at different times. He was brought up in an orphanage and it must have been a struggle for him because he was not physically too robust and was very shortsighted. When I met him he had been Chairman of the Board of Health—he did not wish to be called Health Commissioner—for several years, and although they had changed the Mayor more than once he had remained in office. I believe he remained in charge for some years longer until his health gave way. He had been coroner to the city before taking on the Health Service. I found that out when I went to his office one morning and he threw a newspaper with a picture on it to me. A gangster had been shot. His remark—"One less ! I gave a verdict of murder against him some years ago and he swore he'd get me. He won't now."

One of his favourite stories concerned the arrival of the famous Canadian Dionne quintuplets.

"When I heard about it" he said, "I immediately rang up Dr. Defoe, their medical attendant. When I eventually contacted him after a great deal of difficulty I said to him, ' What you really want is pasteurised human milk, is it not, doctor ?" ' Yes, indeed it is ' he replied. 'I thought as much' I said, 'The plane is on its way with a gallon and there's more available whenever you need it !"

He did much to help public health in that great city, Chicago. The infant mortality rate was one of the lowest in the world, when we in this small country could not believe it was possible. He tackled the problem of the premature baby twenty years before we did. He wiped out diphtheria from the city. One morning in 1943 I was invited to a special meeting of the Board of Health. The members all sat at a round table with Dr. Bundesen in a high chair. He introduced me and the said, "Dr. Parry, the special meeting today is to deal with an outbreak of diphtheria in the Latin Quarter of the city. We have been without the disease for two years. It's a preventable disease ! Of course, I am responsible but I had entrusted the work to Dr. X over there. Jesus Christ had twelve disciples, one of these let him down. What can you expect with Bundesen ?" There was dead silence in the room. I seemed to be the only embarrassed person at the table. But his remedy showed his administrative skill. He had prepared a letter, after consultation with the Archbishop, to be read at all the Roman Catholic Churches in the affected parts. This amounted to an order to all parents to have their children immunised. I did not hear of any further cases of diphtheria in the city after that.

Venereal disease was a great problem in 1943,—especially as several thousand young naval cadets were being trained on Lake Michigan. He discussed the problem with me and said, "I am not concerned with the morals of these young people, but I must keep them healthy. I must therefore keep the women-folk free from disease. I want to write to all the hotels and places frequented by these girls and ask the proprietors to let me have a list of names so that I can have them examined. I have about a hundred social workers available and we can follow up and treat them."

A couple of weeks later on my way back from the Middle West I asked him what had happened to his scheme. He had had several hundred names and a long list that required treatment. Two places only had failed to respond—one ignored him but later came to heel, but the other told him to "go to hell". At once he had the place "posted"—that is cordoned off and posted with notices saying, "Beware. Infectious disease here". A few hours later the last list was to hand. Of course, venereal disease is not classified under the infectious diseases Acts in this country but even if they were what would happen if I did that in Bristol, England ?

I must mention one further example of Dr. Bundesen's self-confidence, courage and ability to make up his mind. He had a report from his sanitary officers, confirmed by laboratory examination, that a certain hotel in the city was lacking in cleanliness in their kitchens. He decided he must act, so he went to the hotel. "I want to see the manager please," he said. "I am afraid he is not in sir. Can I help ? I am the assistant-manager." "Yes, you will do. I am Dr. Bundesen, the Chairman of the Board of Health. From this moment this place is closed as far as serving food is concerned until you have cleaned up your kitchens. The customers here now can finish their meals. You had better say it is closed for alteration and repairs." At once the manager appeared but he could do nothing to persuade the doctor to change his mind. When it was over the manager tried to challenge the law, but I seem to recollect that the doctor won.

I had a very warm corner in my heart for this human dynamo. Nothing was too much trouble for him to do to oblige me and his generous hospitality was so natural and intimate that I could not object. I remember the first time I met him. He arranged to stop the New York train at a Chicago suburban station and there he met me. We were driven to his human milk depot, the first one I had ever seen and it was an eye opener. There, nursing women of all colours and creeds were being milked, after, of course, making quite sure that they were completely healthy. The milk was immediately pasteurized in a special machine on the premises and stored for use for pediatricians to use in hospitals or in the home with particular attention to premature children. The women that supplied the milk were earning ten pounds and more per week—in the days when the pound really was a pound.

Immediately afterwards he took me to the "top" hotel and asked for the manager to whom he introduced me. "And now Mr. Manager", he said, "I don't know what Dr. Parry wants but he must have the best steak you have on the premises, a large ice cream and anything else he wants." I wanted nothing else, alas, because like the rest of British people in the big towns, my stomach was contracted as the result of rationing and I just could not do justice to their wonderful meals. I fared much better in 1951 when he took me to a riverside cafe to a specially prepared meal. That was the last occasion and it was a worthy one. The following morning he came to see me and said

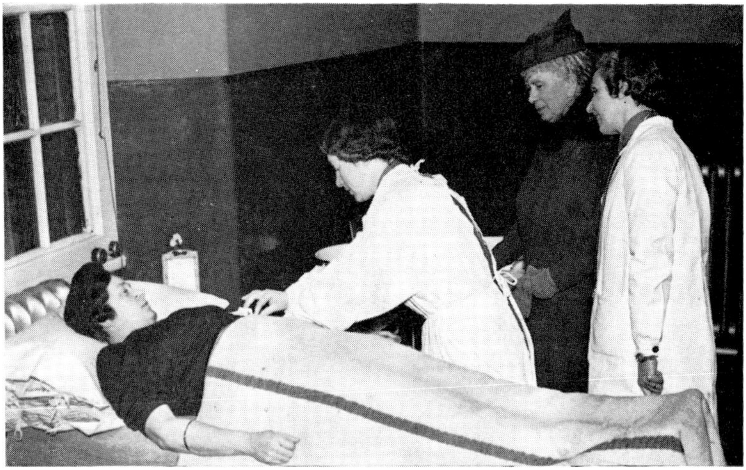

Joan demonstrating the technique of taking blood for transfusion
to Queen Mary during the War

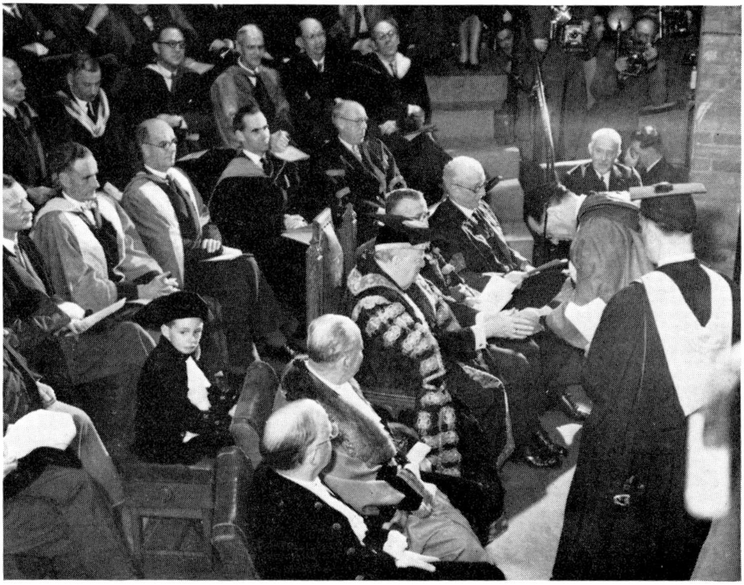

The Chancellor of Bristol University, Mr. Winston Churchill,
conferring degrees after an air raid

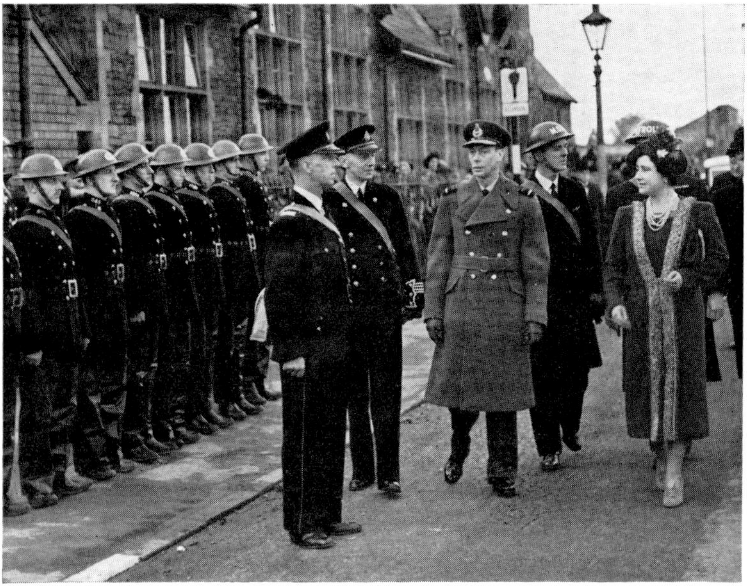

A Royal Visit to Bristol during the blitz

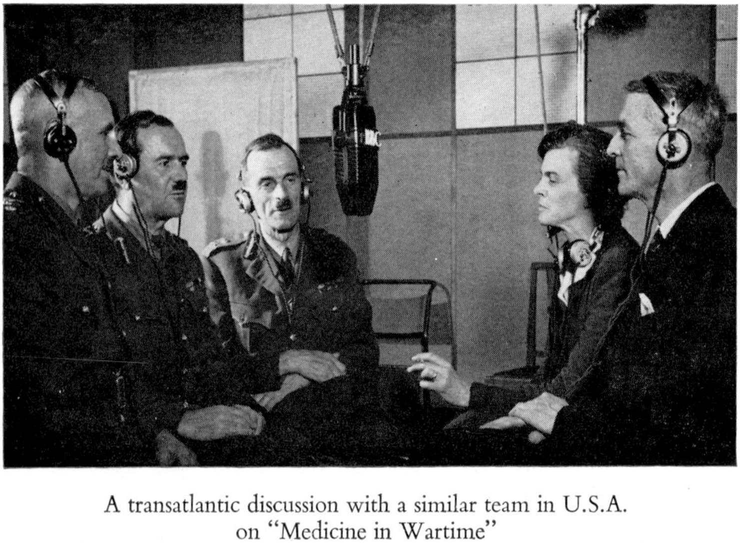

A transatlantic discussion with a similar team in U.S.A. on "Medicine in Wartime"

"Is there anything further you would like to do or see ?" "Yes," I said, "I understand Colonel MacCormac of the Chicago Tribune is very anti-English. I would like to meet him. Perhaps I could recognise the complaint !"

A telephone message followed within a short while—"I will call for you at 2.30 p.m." He did and we proceeded to the Tribune Tower. It was a most useful ride because the doctor gave me a good deal of the background to that powerful press millionaire. We ascended the lift to the ninth floor and were admitted and then handed over our coats and hats and were carefully inspected. Then into the anteroom where there was a man with a couple of hounds on leads—coincidence ? I don't know, and I cannot remember the doctor's remarks but he was not as surprised as I was. Then into the august presence ! A tall, fine-looking man in a tweed suit of plus-fours came forward and the doctor introduced me. The Colonel welcomed me in a quiet, gentle voice.

The conversation went something like this :

"It's very good of you to spare time to see me Colonel, particularly as I understand you are not too fond of us across the water !" He smiled. "What part of Ireland do you hail from—North or South ?"

"The North I suppose."

"In any case you won't particularly like me because a good deal of the trouble in Southern Ireland was caused by exported Welshmen !"

We then talked about his experience in England. He had been to a Buckingham Palace Garden Party and we compared notes. He had thoroughly enjoyed it as a unique experience. It was very obvious that he was just a politician who, like many others, practised what he did not believe. Unfortunately, his political creed was anti-British. I understand that the Tribune Tower is built of stone collected all over the world. As a parting shot I asked him—"You have heard we have lost the Stone of Scone—you don't happen to have it here ? It doesn't really matter, I only wanted a piece as a keepsake." He enjoyed the joke.

Dr. Bundesen congratulated me—"a twenty minute interview is a good deal longer than any I have seen him give." Well ! Well !

Of course, Dr. Bundesen could not have achieved all he did on his income as the Chief Health Executive. His salary at that time in 1943 was twelve thousand dollars a year. He told me he had a private radio service which brought him seventy five thousand a year. Once again we see the advantages of a private income giving that blessed feeling of being independent. He certainly was independent in mind and action. I was told that, on one occasion, when he thought the Mayor of Chicago had obstructed him in some matter of great public health importance he sought an audience of the Mayor and declared bluntly that it could not happen otherwise he would submit his own name as a candidate for the Mayoralty at the next election ! My happy memories of that remarkable man will remain with me for the rest of my life.

There were other interesting events, besides the ones connected with Dr. Bundesen, that occurred to me in Chicago. On May 5th, 1943, I was invited with Dr. Mallon of Toynbee Hall, London, to a dinner party by the British Consul General at the Chicago Club. I remember the date because I have it and the list of guests before me as I write. We were told there would be a total party of twenty including Mr. Gallienne the Consul General, Mr. Thomas the Consul and Mr. Clark of the British Information Services. We were warned we would be expected to say a few words after the dinner. It was indeed a memorable occasion—not only was the dinner well-chosen and a change from our "blitz diet" at home but the invited guests were distinguished Chicagoians and most interesting. One of them, I cannot remember who, was most anxious for me to see the personal telephone service in San Francisco's Chinatown when I was in that city. I understand that you only had to pick up the telephone receiver and ask for a person at an address and immediately you were through. I only wish I had a moment from my busy programme to see this wonder service. Dr. Snyder, the President of North Western University, invited me to address the students in the Library the following morning and it certainly was worth seeing these fine-looking uniformed young men listening attentively to a brief account of our war experience at home.

When I returned to Chicago in 1951 the Consul General arranged a small luncheon party. It started nearly an hour late and I was to catch a train for Ann Arbor in the middle of the afternoon. When I looked at my watch the train must have left an hour before. However, fate came to the rescue, as seemed always to happen to me, when Dr. Maddock, the Professor of Surgery at the North Western University, volunteered to look after me and see me safely installed in time to keep my appointment. He did so by taking me in his car to his flat on Michigan Boulevard. We talked in his bar which was equipped in the style of a South Sea island and then went on to the airport for Detroit.

The person next to me in the plane was being met to be taken to Ann Arbor and I was invited to join him so I arrived sooner than if if I had caught my train.

The other incident in Chicago was most amusing—in 1951. On arriving from Wisconsin I jumped into a taxi at the station to get to the hotel. I had not noticed the driver particularly at first but it seems he had noted me. He was short, tough, Italian-type with a ready smile and we drove along he shouted back to me, "Where you from ?" "Bristol, England". "I can't stop here, there's a cop looking. We'll get a side street." 'What's all this '—said I to myself—' a real hold up ? ' My younger daughter under the dining-table during an air raid once called, "Isn't it exciting—a real air raid !" I must have felt somewhat like that with, maybe, a little more knowledge of what to expect. But I was wrong. "Do you know Filton Laundry ?" "Yes". He tore a slip from his cab and wrote. "Will you go and see the woman in charge and say "Apple-face sends his love. We were stationed in Wiltshire during the war and several times a week I had to take a truck with a load to or from that Laundry. She was so kind to me—like a mother !" I did not succeed, when I returned home, in finding the lady although the press did their best to help.

I addressed several meetings in Chicago during my visit in 1951. One particularly interesting meeting was the Council of Foreign Relations when an old friend whom I knew in Bristol, Mr. Cole, the Canadian Consul, also spoke.

Back to 1943. Part I of the Tour. From Chicago my programme was to Milwaukee and down to the Middle West, Iowa, Kansas (Topeka), Missouri (Jefferson City) and Indiana (Evansville). I was a lone traveller and I could have done with company on some of these journeys although they were most comfortable—to read, eat and sleep. In all these places conferences of some kind were taking place and I joined in the discussion and gave the after-dinner address in the evening. When I arrived at one of these places I felt very bedraggled after a night and a morning in the train. When I was taken to my hotel there were four hours to spare before my programme started so I decided to have my suit pressed and went to bed—having been assured it would be returned well on time. However I started getting restless at 6.30 p.m. and very restless at 7 p.m. because the dinner was at 7.30 p.m. There was consternation in the hotel—the bellboy was off duty. At 7.30 my suit arrived and so did the State Health Commission but I need not have worried because the dinner started at 8.30. That was fairly typical of the unhurried attitude of the very pleasant and hospitable people.

Before the dinner the Health Commissioner and myself had time to turn into the hotel bar to toast each other. He had a good Scottish name—Mac . . . and I proceeded to tell him a few Scottish stories—Always prefixing them with "You Scots are a wonderful people." Without hesitation he relied "Excuse me, doctor, but I am an American." After a few "Old Fashioneds" however his accent became distincly Glaswegian. I persisted with my tactics, hoping to get him to confess that he was a Scot. At last it came—how many old fashioneds it took I know not—but the confession came suddenly when he told a story of how he threatened to strike a notable citizen who had in the heat of the moment stated "You have no right to speak on that subject Dr. Mac . . . because you were born in Glasgow". "And," said he in reply, "the person who dare accuse me of committing a crime by being born in Glasgow is not in this room !" We were both most fluent in our after-dinner speeches !

Milwaukee was a particularly interesting city to me. I visited it twice—in 1943 during my Mid-West tour, and in 1951. In 1943 I was billed to speak after dinner at their annual Tuberculosis Conference. The chairman was the Dean of the Medical School. As we entered the dining-hall a small choir burst into song—the Welsh National Anthem. When I got up to speak I said, "I am delighted to be in Milwaukee for a very personal reason. When I was a very little boy I remember my mother writing to her mother and father in Wisconsin and Milwaukee crept up quite often." I then proceeded with "Tuberculosis in Wartime Britain." When the function was over an elderly white haired little man came up and said, "My name is also Parry—though no relation. May I speak to you doctor ?" "Certainly sir.' "Well, when you were billed to speak here with your Welsh name I made enquiries of the British authorities in New York about your antecedents. I found that I knew your grandfather and grandmother in this country. I was a minister but have been retired many years and am now eithy-four years old. I buried your grandparents and can take you to see their graves if you wish." I am afraid, however, my programme would not permit of my accepting his offer.

After the dinner and my speech were finished we retired into another room for the reception and an opportunity for me to shake hands. Suddenly there stood before me a stocky, plump, short lady with red hair. I remembered her as a girl in the village near where I was born. We said a few words in Welsh to each other and she burst into tears of homesickness and vanished. Eight years later I was billed to speak again in Milwaukee. This time it was on civil defence and I recognised the German discipline of the guard-of-honour of civil defence workers and nurses as led by the Mayor with the Chief Constable and Civil Defence Chief as we marched onto the platform in the City Hall. The large hall was packed. The Mayor made his introduction and I stepped up the large platform on to the microphone. As I looked down on the audience, there in the centre of the front row with her handkerchief at the ready was the little lady of eight years ago.

In 1943 during part of my tour I went to Boston, Massachusetts and I enjoyed my visit very much. My first engagement was a dinner with Dr. Claire Turner, the great authority on health education at the Mass. Institute of Technology. It was a delightful start and introduction to Boston. The following day I was to speak at the Colloquiem at Harvard at lunchtime. A small party of medical professors and the Dean of the Faculty accompanied me and when we had consumed our repast one of the professors stood up to introduce me to the gathering. He enumerated the different members of the "Parry" family who had served U.S.A. well—quite a lesson to me. After such high praise it was not for me to disclaim relationship ! But alas it was all new to me. In fact when I visited Lincoln Nebraska a few weeks later the newspaper announced Sir Hubert Parry as a visitor—for the rest of my journeys with the party I was known as Sir Hubert although I warned them I might be a Duke before we finished. One lady in the same city said she had enjoyed the company of Lady Hamilton the previous year. My facetious enquiry about Nelson was wasted ! At the Colloquiem, however, I was able to thank the Medical School for sending the Harvard Unit stationed at Salisbury under Dr. John Gordon over to Bristol to help us clear up a big epidemic of paratyphoid.

I then had a luncheon engagement at the Harvard Club and spoke a few words before Dr. Agnes Hamilton the great pioneer in industrial medicine. And what a charming and wonderful lady she was. She was a fluent, easy speaker. With all those qualities no wonder she was such a great influence in the development of industrial medicine in her country.

Dr. Dwight O'Hara then took charge of me. He was a descendant of the Boston Irish and I have a feeling he was anxious to tell me how Boston put the English in their place. When, however, he discovered I was Welsh although in a way he was disappointed he took me to his home and introduced me to his lady who was a former pupil at the Red Maids School in Bristol. Dr. O'Hara, an epidemiologist of the first rank, (I have before me a most useful book by him on the subject) was Dean of the Medical Faculty of Tufts Medical School. Whilst we were resting, waiting for our dinner engagement, a small forest fire occurred a few yards from the house. It was soon put out but it did give me an idea of the danger that lies in dry climates if forest fires should break out. Indeed I do not think this country appreciates the damage done to human beings and to material things by smoking. It is surprising that insurance companies do not load the premiums where smoking is permitted. Of course, non-smokers are to blame for not insisting on special insurance rates or establishing more companies to cater for them because now they are charged extra for the damage done by smoking !

In the evening I spoke after dinner at the Harvey Society of Tufts and the students' president made me a member of the Honour Society Alpha Omega Alpha.

In 1951 I was invited back to Tufts to give the address at the opening of the New England Medical Centre. It really was in advance of anything I had seen in this country—its large dental training school was on a grand scale and had the latest equipment. The meeting on this occasion was in one of the lecture-rooms and broadcast by loud-speakers to other lecture-halls. When I arrived home in Bristol I found three aluminium discs of all the proceedings—an interesting keepsake for the family. It was amusing to be introduced to an audience in Boston as an Honorary Physician to the King of England ! A tea party in reverse. Later on Dr. Grace, a well-known surgeon from New York, arranged to take me to see the Business School at Harvard and I attended a class. It was beyond me really, but I do appreciate that it would be possible to grow up to it ! In the evening he gave a private dinner-party and when he was toasting his guest I suddenly remembered it was the anniversary of my wedding day.

At once two more bottles of champagne were ordered. It was as well I was staying at the hotel that night !

Back again to 1943. I went to John Hopkins Medical School in Baltimore and met many of the staff whom afterwards I claimed amongst my best friends among them Dr. Huntingdon Williams, the Health Commissioner. I spoke to him again on the transatlantic radio from the B.B.C. in September 1943 when three military doctors and myself as a civilian and a similar number of American military doctors with Dr. Huntingdon Williams and with Alistair Cooke in the chair and Mary Adams as our chairman. I have now some aluminium discs of our discussion on "Medicine in Wartime"—a real treasure, for it was the first of its kind undertaken by the B.B.C. On my arrival in Baltimore I was taken to address a class on health education and afterwards met some famous people including Sigerist, the medical historian, and Dr. MacCallum, the authority on vitamins.

It was most interesting to meet these great men who had been mere names to me. Sigerist's books on the history of medicine had always thrilled me and I treasure a booklet he gave me on "The importance of health to a city" written by a German author and edited by himself. I listened with interest to Dr. MacCallum's account of his early pioneering days in investigating vitamins. He was amused when I asked him if he knew the origin of the word ' Vitamines ' and confessed he had never thought of it. I then told him this story :—

Dr. Nierenstein, a colleague in the University of Bristol, a reader in Biochemistry and the greatest authority on the chemistry of colour, was a good friend of mine and we often discussed medical and non-medical matters. Dr. Funk, a pioneer in vitamine research, had a private laboratory in Paris and on several occasions came over to Bristol to discuss his problems with Nierenstein. He was convinced that colour in some way was associated with certain vitamines. Usually he arrived in Bristol at the week-end but for no-one would Nierenstein sacrifice his Saturday game of golf. So, on this particular occasion, Funk joined him. Now if you had seen Nierenstein you would have realised at once that he could not possibly be a great golfer because of his physique. Besides, his temperament was not suitable as he was, like many of us, quick-tempered. On the 17th tee at Henbury golf course he had missed his drive—thirty yards only—and as he was taking his second shot Funk came along and proceeded to continue expounding his theories on the ' accessory food factors ' (or as he pronounced it 'acthethary food factorth,' for he lisped badly). Nierenstein missed his second shot, dropped his golf bag and let fly. His full speech is not recorded but he made it clear to Funk that some word or words that he could pronounce clearly would be 'less annoying'. If he thought they were 'amines' chemically and were necessary to life why not call them 'Vitamines'. When Dr. Funk returned to Paris he wrote to Nierenstein saying that he liked the term and would use it forthwith. That historic letter could still be in existence. Dr. MacCallum jumped up, left the room and returned with his monograph on Vitamines. In a note at the bottom of a page were the words that the term Vitamine was first used by Funk. He was delighted with the story and made full notes of it.

The same story, much abbreviated, caused great amusement at the Bristol Rotary Club on one occasion. Professor Hirst of the University was giving an after-lunch talk on Vitamines on which he was an authority. In reply to questions from the chairman I stood up and said "Fellow Rotarians, you will be interested to know that the term 'Vitamine' was invented on the 17th fairway of Henbury Golf Course. It's a long story which I may tell you one day." The Evening Papers had little to say about the fine address by Professor Hirst but the headlines blazed "Vitamines invented on Henbury golf course". What makes news !

The tour of the Western States was organised by the American Public Health Association under the leadership of Dr. Atwater, the Secretary. There were twelve of us in the team. We started in New York with a conference and a dinner at which I spoke—the chairman was Dr. Bristol which augured well for the tour ! Chicago, Nebraska, Denver Colorado—the mile high city—Albuquerque, Phoenix Arizona, Los Angeles, San Francisco, Portland Oregon, Seattle, Boise Idaho, and then by myself to Salt Lake City. At most of these places something unexpected and usually amusing occurred and I have already mentioned some of these. I would now like to mention a few more because they give me 'food for thought' and an insight into other people's point-of-view.

At the conference in Lincoln, Nebraska, health-workers were complaining of the lack of doctors in the rural areas and small towns. We had a housing estate in Bristol and there was considerable agitation lest the people should suffer because the nearest doctor lived over a mile away. In Nebraska it was somewhat different—some settlements of several thousand people had a distance of over two hundred miles to get to the nearest doctor! I took this message home to Bristol to cheer them up.

In Denver, Colorado, they had approximately seven wet days a year and plenty of sunshine. After one meeting a lady came to me and asked if I could do anything to get her home to England. I said "Where in England?" "Liverpool." I said, "Make the most of this sunshine. You will get little of it when you return to Liverpool". "I know," she said very severely, "But it is my home".

In Phoenix, Arizona, two incidents occurred. In the hall of the hotel a man approached me and presented his card. He was a rodent operator and doing very well—but he wanted to let me know he was still British although he would rather I did not spread the information for business reasons! On the first morning I was roused at 6.30 a.m. by the telephone and a man's voice said there was a combined British-American air-training camp about ten miles out and it was graduation day—would I care to come along? I said yes and a stranger picked me up and drove me to the air-station. We were too late for the ceremony but the commanding officer was a flying doctor from Scotland. His father was still in practice there—would I give him a message when I got back? I did so. I met two young Bristol boys who had just finished their training. Next year I had a note from the doctor from a Wiltshire camp. When the war was over he wrote again to say that he had settled down in Phoenix in practice as a doctor.

In Los Angeles I met Mrs. Howard Hutter and there rests a good story. I considered Howard as one of my best friends; we had got on so well together in Bristol but I had not yet, of course, met his wife. He had written to her to tell her I was coming over. One day in New York I had a wire "Looking forward to seeing you. Diana." In Chicago, "Feel I know you already. Good wishes. Diana." When we arrived at the Baltimore Hotel in Los Angeles there was another message, "As soon as you arrive ring up this number please. Welcome. Diana." I rang up the number and spoke to Diana. "Stay in the hall and I will call for you." "How shall I know you?" (I did not then know that she was from the Philipines). "I shall wear a tall black hat." I waited in an osbcure corner of the hall and every lady that came in had a black hat! Presently, however, a lovely lady with a lovely cape and a tall, Welsh type, hat entered and my name was called. I nearly collapsed. What would my companions say?—they knew not of the

Hutters ! In no time we were in a cab and so to the Athletic Club for a good lunch. The following day she introduced us to Miss Meyer at the Metro Goldwyn Meyer Studios and we were shown round to see some of the actors at work—Robert Taylor, Fay Baynter, Red Skelton, and Diana herself was playing a leading part in a film.

We saw a good deal of the Hutters when my wife and I visited the U.S.A. in 1951 and 1956. On both occasions we attended a reception in their lovely home in Long Island. Their home was a bungalow fitted with furniture from the Philipinnes. We were interviewed by the press and met many of their friends. On the second occasion a lady singer brought with her her own little organ and we had a concert and Diana herself danced. There was always a great welcome for us and both our eldest son and our younger daughter have spent enjoyable week-ends in their fine home.

Still in 1943, for the first time in my life I went with the party to a large self-service restaurant. There were six long counters on both sides. My plates were filled before I had cleared four sides out of the twelve and I had to ask if I could start again with empty plates !

On our last evening in Los Angeles, Miss Denning and I had to address the District Nurses Association. They had six full-time nurses. Our Clifton and Bristol District Nurses Association, of which I was Honorary President, had thirty-five at that time so I could speak with conviction about their value in a community. We then went to a private dinner-party and rushed by cab to catch our train for San Francisco.

It was a pleasure to meet my friends in San Francisco and I was delighted to see Dr. Geiger, the Health Commissioner at the dinner for he had not been on good terms with the American Public Health Association. Maybe that was my good deed for the day. When I had visited San Francisco in 1935 the big bridge across the bay to Berkeley had not been built. Now the bridges were completed and we were able to visit in comfort the great red woods across the bay. We stayed in a beautiful hotel in Berkeley and I was welcomed especially with a bouquet of flowers. San Francisco has often been called the Bristol of the West Coast—but it is on a much grander scale than the old city in England. They had just discovered some British coins and other evidence buried by Captain Cook that proved he had been there.

When I reached Portland Oregon, I experienced an example of American generosity. I had been given a daily allowance by the British Information Services during my visit and this would not have gone very far. But the American hospitality was such that I had not exhausted this allowance. However, when I arrived in Portland there was a package waiting for me. It was from the Rockfeller Foundation and it contained a handsome book of dollar cheques with a note "Please use as you wish—we are afraid your allowance is rather meagre—all we ask is that you fill in the counterfoils." I think I used only one—the need did not arise.

One other memory of this city of roses and sea foods—I found a small pearl in a large oyster and have kept it as a keepsake of my visit to Portland Oregon.

In Seattle, another great city, we were able to visit the lovely home of a 'lumber king' on the other side of the bay. What wealth and what beautiful homes in such lovely surroundings.

Seattle is the Capital of Washington State on the West coast bordering on British Columbia. I was to speak after dinner at an Annual Conference and the following somewhat amusing incident took place.

We were just sitting down to dinner—I was between the President of the Conference and the British Consul General—a young man from an English Public School—when I noticed a man and a lady walking to their seat a little late. Instantly, as fate sometimes steps in, I remembered having seen them in my home, Penllwyn, many years ago. Their name was Griffiths and Mrs. Griffiths was a professional singer. We stood up to sing "The Star Spangled Banner" and then "God Save the King." I turned to the President and said "It is very good of you to sing the English National Anthem in my honour but it isn't really my national anthem. There was considerable rustling on my right and I could visualise the British Consul seeing the British Empire going to hell—this was long before it did ! "Oh Doctor, isn't it—I thought you were English." I said "No, I am Welsh and our National Anthem is "Hen Wlad fy Nhadau". "What do we do now ?" said the President. "If you are interested" I replied, "I have seen Mrs. Griffiths among the diners ; perhaps she would sing it ?" The President called for order, told my story and asked if Mrs. Griffiths would oblige. She said she would be delighted. She went to the piano and we all stood up for the third time and she and I sang "Hen Wlad fy Nhadau" in Welsh !

And so to Boise, Idahó. There we had a parting dinner prepared by Dr. McCowan in a country club. He supervised the serving as well wearing his chef cap. A small presentation was made to Dr. Atwater, who had been such a wonderful guide, philosopher, friend and master of ceremonies at our meetings especially "The brains' trusts" which were put on at some places. I was presented with a cowboy hat and a silk scarf!

We parted company here, for me to go to Salk Lake City, the city of the Mormons. There I felt very much at home. The Mayor -Ap Jenkins, was a racing motorist, the Health Commissioner was Dr. Howell and the State Health Commissioner Dr. MacKay was a brother of the Chief Mormon and had learned to speak Welsh from his mother. What a wonderful city it is; surrounded by snowclad mountains and all roads leading to the Mormon Tabernacle. We were fortunate when we went to the Church to find the organist looking round and he played for us. It is built very much like Epidaurus in Greece with stage and organ at the bottom and not an echo anywhere. What a pity the experts who advised on the building of the old senate room in Bristol University had not visited it to learn something about acoustics.

Impressions of the tour by members of the party were printed in the American Public Health Journal of July 1943. My travelling companions were specially selected for an experiment in wartime decentralisation. They were not only experts in their own subjects but national figures in that great country. Much of the glory was reflected onto their sole foreign guest and their comments were too generous in their tribute to the part I played.

During the tour of the public health team through the Western States, which was indeed both a test and an examination, it became my responsibility, as the foreign guest to give the 'after dinner' address at each State conference—some dozen or more. I enjoyed most the discussion by the team, usually in the train perparatory to the meetings. My companions went as far as to suggest the stories that suited the territory best from among my collection. Of course, as they pointed out, there were long distances between the different state capitals and there was no reason whatsoever for not repeating the same speech! I was deeply impressed at one of these earlier dinners when I found several of my colleagues sitting in and listening to my repeated "sermons". When I expressed my appreciation and apologies for the repetition they soon dissilusioned me by saying that they could not get out in time without showing extreme discourtesy! They were prepared for this contingency at future dinners. I was delighted really with their strategy for there would remain, now, no-one who could collect and repeat extracts from my many speeches. However, I was mistaken. When Dr. Albert McCown, Director of the American Red Cross and a member of the team, came over to Britain he visited us in Bristol. He wrote a letter which was published in the American Journal of Public Health summarising my speeches. I have permission from the executive director, Dr. Berwyn F. Mattison, to use it :—

Excerpts from Dr. McCown's Letter
Director of the American Red Cross Organisation

"I went down to Bristol on the Saturday morning train, arriving in time for lunch, stayed over Sunday, made some official visits Monday morning, and returned Monday afternoon.

I cannot tell you what a satisfaction it was to see Dr. Parry in his home environment. His wife is a charming person, a Captain in the British Medical Corps, doing a splendid job in the transfusion service. I shall not attempt to describe their home; their gardens; their friends; nor the place they occupy in the life of Bristol. You will have to come and see it for yourself, and I do hope that some day you will have that privilege.

The purpose of this letter is to confirm for you and the other members of the troupe the accuracy of Dr. Parry's description of Bristol, as immortalized in the famous opus we heard on so many occasions.

First of all, of course, I saw the famous River Avon, down which some famous journeys were made. John Cabot, among others, sailing out to discover a new world, not forgetting that one of the promoters of that voyage was the Sheriff of Bristol, a Mr. Americke. Dr Parry insists that "whatever the Italians say, we in Bristol know that that was the origin of the word America."

Bristol is a City of Churches, mostly burnt out now, built with money made out of the slave trade, a sort of Beveridge scheme for the next world. Now, in the year of our Lord 1944, we find that Bristol's gift of slaves is being returned to Bristol with interset.

I saw, too, St. Mary's, Redcliff, which Queen Elizabeth said was the most beautiful Parish Church in England, and so it must be, because no one has ever dared to disagree with Queen Elizabeth !

Sunday afternoon we drove up the road to Cheddar, through the rocky Combe of Barrington, where the Vicar of Blagdon, the Rev. A. M. Toplady, caught in a storm of thunder, lightning and torrential rain found refuge in a cleft in the rocks, and, as a result of that experience, wrote the hymn, "Rock of Ages, Cleft for me, Let me hide myself in thee."

On the way back we passed the quay-side of the Port of Bristol, immortalized by Robinson Crusoe and John Silver, and on past the site where St. Peter's hospital used to be, and where worked William Budd, the father of epidemiology. I saw no statue to Jenner. Undoubtedly this would not nave been permitted by the anti-vaccinationists, since Bristol is their headquarters. I saw the little brick "cottages"—with their amenities. (Just between you and me they are really two story brick houses but the Bristolians insist on calling them cottages, and cottages they must remain.)

From without, I worshipped at the Chapel of John Wesley, the Founder of Wesleyism and saw the Castle stormed by Sir Thomas Fairfax during the Cromwellian period. It was the same Fairfax family who figured so largely in early American history, it being a Lord Fairfax who owned tremendous estates in Virginia surveyed by a youthful George Washington.

In Dr. Parry's own home I saw a Morrison style shelter, just as he had described it. Fortunately there was no necessity to use it during my visit.

So completely delightful was the trip, and so wholehearted the welcome, that Hugh Smith and I plan to go down for another week-end in the near future."

It is really very difficult to imagine U.S.A. as one country and one nation. Yet, patriotism exuded from everyone wherever we went. It was expressed somewhat differently in the different states and I understand some of their laws were very different. I only came across this once when I decided it was time that I had a party in my room. I found great difficulty in finding the necessary "bottles" but they did appear after much stimulating of the hotel staff. When my party met they protested vigorously that I had waited until we reached the capital of a "dry state" before giving the party ! However, it did not affect the happiness of the occasion. It was a great experience to visit the West and we all often quoted a poem which was repeated so often on the train as we travelled west that in the end we could swear it was true ! "Out where the West begins . . ."

I am writing this in 1969—twenty six years later. Young men have gone west which has now a vastly increased population. I wonder if all this change has altered the theme of the poem ?

Still in 1943, part three of my visit was sponsored by the Rockefeller Foundation. I visited institutions and personalities connected with public health. In New York City at Columbia University I met that great person, Dr. Haven Emerson, a nephew of the essayist. He had been Health Commissioner for New York and was now partly retired but helping at Columbia. During my 1951 visit I was privileged, with my wife and Dr. and Mrs. Darling, to visit him on his estate in Long Island and meet him and Mrs. Emerson in their home surroundings. And what a home !—complete with boat and slip to Long Island Sound ! Every item of food at the lunch had been prepared by Dr. Emerson himself. Before many months I had the sad task of writing a note to the Lancet after his death. Public Health owes much to his pioneering efforts and his dauntless courage in advocating change. Amongst his schemes was the fluoridation of water which he advocated strongly as the result of scientific investigation.

A visit to East Harlem health-centre was an eye-opener. Let us remember this was twenty six years ago and there was a war on !

But this little health-centre looked after the public health and clinical needs of a vast population. The senior physician in charge was a Russian doctor. Her people in the area were roughly 20% negro, 27% Puerto Rican who are incensed at being called coloured and who hate the Italians, and about 25% Italian and 25% poor Europeans. What a problem to solve ! They mostly lived in tenement dwellings or old multi-storied houses and many a family in one room. I still believe that the solution lies in new towns for these people, with good homes and good industries and self-government and the coloured people themselves are also beginning to think so too.

It was during this visit that I met Mayor La Guardia, that dynamic and famous administrator of New York. He had three disqualifications as far as the electors were concerned—he was half Italian, half Jew and he was a Non-Conformist in religion. The Health Commissioner, Professor Stebbings, took me to see him one day to hear them discussing the Health estimates for the year. The Mayor convinced me then that government is the job of trained, properly qualified experts. The control of these experts is a separate issue but in this country we have confused the two aspects.

The Mayor told me the following good story. The Chief of Hospitals for New Yorks was retiring after a long and efficient service. The Mayor sent for him to thank him on behalf of the people of New York for his great service. "Before you go, Doctor, could you tell me if you have anybody in mind to succeed you ?" "No" said the doctor, "I really can't say that I know of anybody, but I do hope the man who takes up the post will have private means". "I am amazed" said the mayor, "that you who have always been so forward-looking that your only suggestion for your successor is that he should have private means. What on earth are you thinking about ?" "Well," said the doctor, "I repeat, I hope he has private means but of course that should not be his only qualification. Whenever I have come to see you I have told you quite clearly what I had in mind and cared little about your reactions because I was not dependent on my salary for my way of life."

This story is a great lesson—as the Scottish National Poet has put it :

> "Gather gear in every way . . .
> It gives one the blessed feeling of being independent."

On another occasion Mayor La Guardia sent one of his staff to take me to see Bristol Basin with the plaque on the side of the bridge worded as follows :—

"Beneath this East River Drive of the City of New York lie stones, bricks and rubble from the bombed City of Bristol in England. Brought her in ballast from overseas, these fragments that once were homes shall testify while men love freedom to the resolution and fortitude of the people of Britain. They saw their homes struck down without warning . . . it was not their walls but their valor that kept them free . . .

And broadbased under all is planted England's oaken hearted mood, as rich in fortitude as e'er went worldward from the island wall."

The Mayor gave me a photograph of the plaque and of the Basin for the Lord Mayor of Bristol and a copy for myself.

In Ann Arbor Medical School I had a particularly warm welcome under the kindly wing of Dr. and Mrs. Henry Vaughan, the Dean of the Public Health School. He had previously been Health Commis-

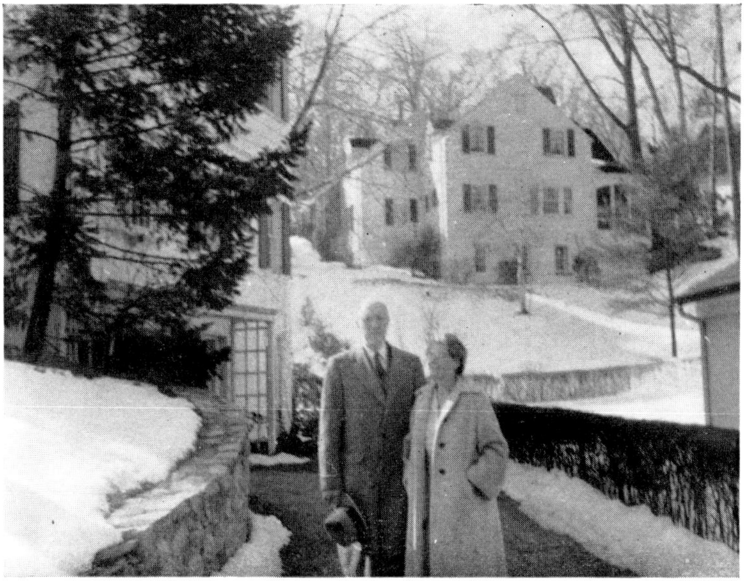

Dr. and Mrs. Reg Atwater outside their home in Bronxsville. He was Secretary to the American Public Health Association

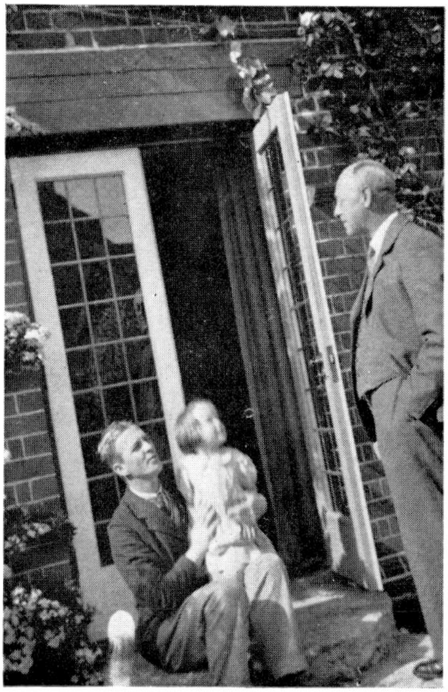

Discussing golf (?) with Professor W. W. Jameson

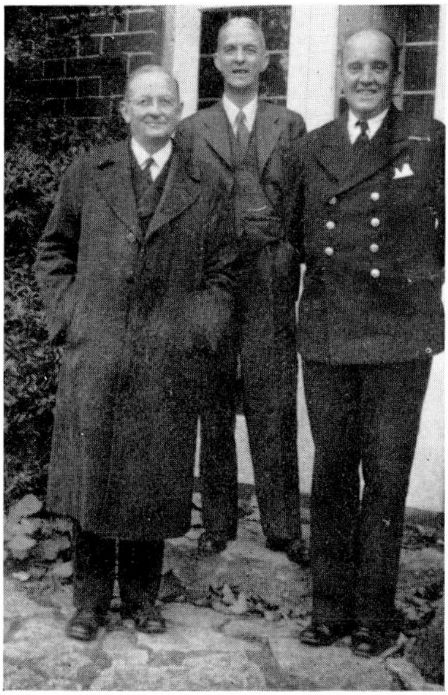

Dr. Charles Best of insulin fame and Dr. Little on a visit to Bristol (1940)

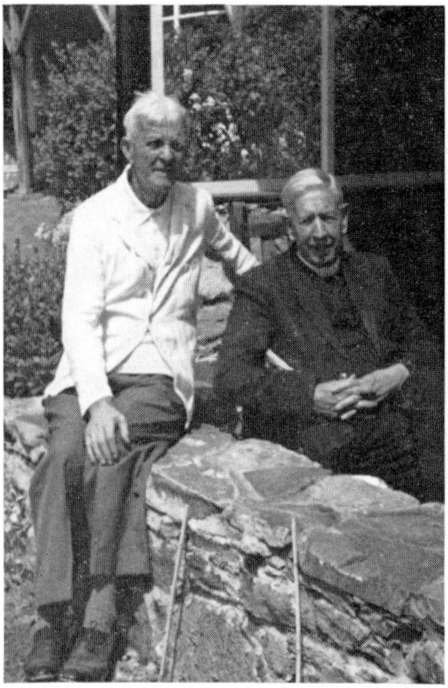

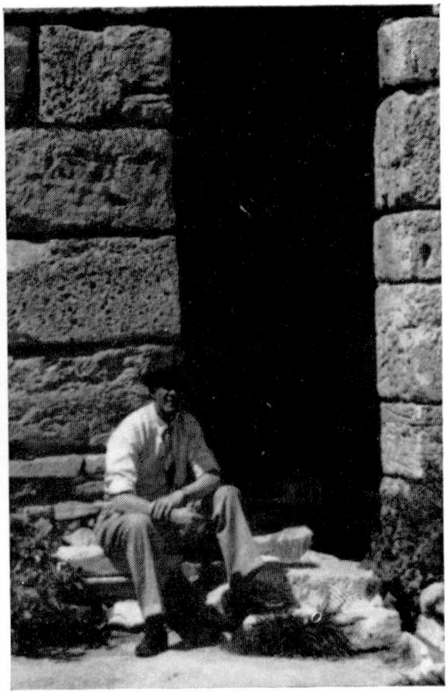

With Canon Gethin Jones during his annual visit to Cefniwrch

At the Sanctuary of Aescalypius on the side of the Acropolis, Athens

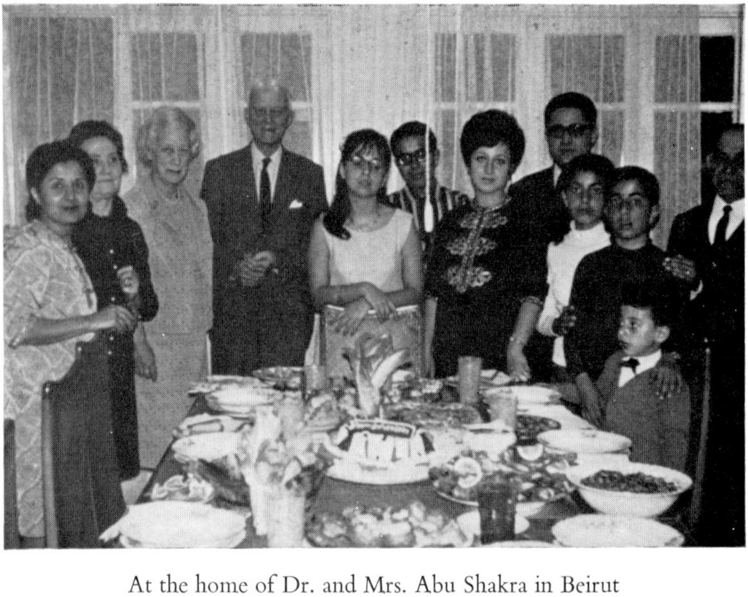

At the home of Dr. and Mrs. Abu Shakra in Beirut celebrating the forty-fourth anniversary of our wedding

sioner of Detroit and was well-known throughout the United States as an outstanding administrator. The University Hospital had established its military wing with the American First Army in Frenchay Hospital, Bristol, and it was great fun to bring messages from their husbands to a gathering of the wives ! Alas, I gave the show away ! for they did not know where in England their husbands were stationed as this was a military secret. We still have many friends in Ann Arbor where we called again in 1956.

Vanderbilt University in Tennessee, where I spent three days in very hot weather, I found most interesting. Here there was a research project, fostered by the Rockefeller Foundation, into the influence of heredity upon tuberculosis. A stable community going back at least one hundred and fifty years gave them the opportunity for field research. Here I met Dr. Bird, a Medical Adviser and Director of a big insurance company. He said his only son, a doctor, was in the army stationed near Bristol and I gave him my address.

I decided I just could not stay in that heat for the week-end so arranged to travel back by air to New York on the Saturday afternoon. I was seated in the plane when, lo, with four other passengers, I was turned off the plane for V.I.P. army personnel. I went to the counter and spoke to the clerk who apologised and said I could be their guest at the Andrew Jackson Hotel and they would take me to New York as soon as they could but that I had no priority. "What does that mean and how can I get it ?" I asked. I was told that for this plane-service I had to ring Memphis so I enquired the name and 'phone number. The girl on the exchange said "One hour's delay". "But you can't do that" I said, "this is urgent". She then put me straight through to the person in charge. "Hello" I said, "This is Dr. Parry from England speaking. I have had priority to cross the Atlantic, could I have priority to go on the next plane from Nashville to New York ?" "Certainly, Doctor" came the reply, "We will arrange your transport and your seat at midnight on the next plane". And so it was.

I wonder if this could ever happen in England even after filling in several forms in triplicate ? Nevertheless, by losing the first plane I lost the opportunity of being Mayor La Guardia's guest at a "Ball Game" which it was his custom to attend on Sunday mornings. He had been trying to find me.

Some weeks later, after I had returned home, I received a telephone call from Dr. Bird Junior in camp a mere ninety miles from Bristol! He came over to see us but it took him nearly all day and he had to be "taken ill" and phone his unit to stay until the following day. In the meantime we had an evening at the Bristol Savages together.

I went on another visit to Nashville in 1951, arranged by Dr. Bird. Dr. Bird Junior, although in the American Parachute Regiment, did arrive safely back home when the war was over.

Dr. Bird had arranged for me to address the Faculty of Medicine in Vanderbilt University and to attend a reception and dinner after. At the reception a fine specimen of a man came towards me. He was 6 ft. 6 ins. tall, broad-shouldered and with penetrating blue eyes, Dr· Hugh Morgan, Professor of Medicine. Our conversation went something like this :—

"I am delighted to meet you, Dr. Morgan—I believe you were the General who was chief consultant to the American Army during the war." "Yes," he replied. "I particularly like your name 'Morgan'—like Parry, a good Welsh name. He said he was descended from the Welsh and proceeded to tell me the following story. "I was on tour of inspection and entered an Officers Mess in a Nissen hut and as I was walking along an officer came quickly towards me and said "Is your name Morgan?" (he had taken no notice of my rank) and I answered "Yes, but I do not know you." "No, Sir" he replied, "I have never met you, but in civilian life I am a Professor of History and am just completing a book on the life of Henry Morgan, the bucaneer, and when I saw you I said to myself, 'if that man only had face cover he would be the image of the famous buccaneer'. "Well I can tell you" I replied, "that it is a tradition in our family that we are descended from a buccaneer and that my grandfather's name was Henry".

"Thank you Dr. Morgan" I said, "that is a lovely story. Like Henry Morgan I am a Bristol Welshman though not yet a buccaneer May I tell the story to the Bristol City Fathers?" "Certainly, it's all yours" he said.

I had often wondered why nurses could not be trained like medical students and be free to attend classes and lectures and to be tied to a period of ward practice. Of course this could be done but up to the present time our old-fashioned method has been cheap labour to the people running the institutions. Propaganda called the profession a "vocation" in the same way that clergy of all denominations are kept in penury. The head of the Nursing School in Vanderbilt had worked out a scheme for nurses training on these lines and the hospitals were staffed with a basic staff of trained nurses and orderlies, independent of the pupil nurses who were attached at various stages for practice. I am convinced that such a method will ultimately prove both more efficient and more economic. Of course, the time is never opportune to change!

In 1943 I returned from the United States through Toronto to Montreal and thence by Liberator to Prestwick. I understand this was the first time, after Mr. Churchill's, that a Liberator had comfortable seating fitted. It certainly was much more comfortable than my journey to the States. However, it took longer to get from Prestwick to Bristol than to Prestwick from Montreal though I found a plane to take me to Hendon.

In 1943 I did meet some interesting and, at that time, well-known pressmen and found them most stimulating—Quentin Reynolds and Robert Bingham being, of course, outstanding. They wanted me to give my impressions of the country before I left but they were not at all clear to me at the time—the impressions came to me later when I had time to think. When I told the City Council my impressions following my 1951 visit they really confirmed the imprints on my memory of the previous visit.

In 1951 I was again approached by the British Information Services to visit U.S.A. This time the request came from the New York Welsh Society. They complained that they were always sending Scotsmen to address Burns Society but never a Welshman on St. David's Day! There was almost a simultaneous invitation from Tufts Medical School in Boston for me to give the oration on the occasion of the opening of the New England Medical Centre at Boston. This time I was not so excited at the thought of going although it would be a pleasure to meet many old friends once again. My wife kept me company and we travelled by the *Queen Mary*. My first excitement, of course, was my engagement to speak after dinner at the Waldorf Astoria to the Welsh Society on St. David's Day. But as we were getting ready to go we were rushed to the television studio to be interviewed and give a short greeting in Welsh to the audience. I am now becoming inured to surprises. The first person I saw at the Waldorf was a little white haired lady whom I recognised as the young pupil teacher from a little village school in Wales. It was she who had received me into that school just over fifty years before. And indeed that is how I started my talk. The other speaker was Sir Gladwyn

Jebb, a border county man, who was then representing this country in U.N.O.

I think I am right in saying that in that great city of New York is the largest Chapel organisation in the world. I refer to the Riverside Chapel. When it was being built by Mr. J. D. Rockefeller Jun. with a blank cheque he decided to ask Dr. Harry Fosdick, a Baptist Minister, in New York, if he would become its chief minister (I think there were at least seven other ministers) and to state his terms. A week later Mr. Rockefeller had a letter refusing his offer. He asked for an appointment to see Dr. Fosdick and the conversation went somewhat like this :—

"Why do you refuse, Dr. Fosdick ? It must be non-denominational but, apart from that condition, just state your own terms." "It's nothing to do with that" said Dr. Fosdick. "Have you ever thought what people would think of me, a minister, if I become associated with you, a millionaire ?" "I see" said Mr. Rockefeller, "and have you thought what people will think of me, a millionaire, if I become associated with you, a minister of religion ?" A week later Dr. Fosdick accepted the post.

I was staying the week-end with a friend, Dr. Atwater, who lived just outside New York City. On the Saturday afternoon he took me to a Garden Party given by the Riverside Chapel and I was privil-edged to spend some time with Dr. Fosdick who had just retured from being the Senior Minister.

Dr. Fosdick relates a very good story from his early life. His father was walking down the garden path one morning to catch the bus to his office, and his mother was standing by the door seeing him off. He stepped and called to her "Mary, tell Harry to cut the grass today if he feels like it"—and then, as an afterthought, "and tell him he had better feel like it !"

Dr. Fosdick tells that this little episode influenced his life very much. When he had a job to do—pleasant or unpleasant—his father's words would come back to him and he tried to approach the job "feeling like it".

An incident occurred on the Sunday I went to the Riverside Chapel which I think is worth recording. I was accompanying Dr. Atwater and as we stepped into the crowded aisle on our way out my friend turned to a small man and said, "Mr. J. D. Rockefeller Junior, meet Dr. Parry from Wales". "And what part of Wales do you come from ?" "From Criccieth" said I. "Well", he said, "I know Criccieth well. I cycled through Criccieth". "On a push bike ?" I asked. "Yes, on a push bike" replied the millionaire !

General MacArthur came to New York the day after making his famous speech of resignation in Washington. A friend had invited me to lunch at a Bank restaurant in Wall Street. When I met him he politely told me that an "English" accent was not too popular in New York at that moment and it was much too serious a moment for joking. I took his hint and listened carefully. Little was said but the feeling was intense, tears were frequent and the anti-British feeling was terrific. The trouble is that maybe I was carried away by my contacts, especially one of my best friends, Dr. Hutter, the personal doctor of General MacArthur, but my sympathies were very much on the side of the General.

During this shorter visit I travelled quickly and visited fifteen universities, lecturing at twelve of them—usually on the National Health Services and what it meant to the people of Britain. This was not a popular subject to the medical fraternity—some even going as far as to suggest that we were misusing the Marshall Aid. However, I had many old friends who stood firm and insisted I was only telling them what was happening not what I thought.

The tour started with a visit to Washington for a lunch with the Director General of Medical Services and from there went, at my own request, to see the Tennessee Valley administration. This was the greatest state-venture of its kind in the world. The purpose was to control the waters of the Tennessee River which opens into the Ohio and then into the Mississippi. Thereby an enormous area of waste land was irrigated and developed, free electricity was developed and swamps which caused much malaria were destroyed. This really shows what a country can do if it wants to do it.

Then to Atlanta City and a visit to the golf course of the famous Bobbie Jones. Need I say it ?—wonderful ! In the club house are the four golf balls with which Bobbie Jones completed his rounds which won the four world championships—amateur and professional in America and Britain.

We were invited to a delightful tea party in Atlanta at an old colonial mansion on the outskirts of the town. In the spacious dining room our hostess poured out tea for the ladies at one end of the dining table while our host dispensed buorbon for those men-folk who were not accustomed to afternoon tea. Our hostess told us that the lovely silver tea-service she was using had been buried by a faithful old coloured servant during the Civil War to save it from being looted and that the grandson of the old negro was still in their service.

Down to Jacksonville, Florida, where we had several surprises. It was snowing there and some had never seen snow in that city. It soon cleared up. I there met Mr. Roosevelt's medical attendant, whose name has escaped me, who had passed him fit for his last term as President. He has, of course, been much criticised but, after all, he was only a doctor and not a prophet. He was an interesting person with a good sense of humour and a fund of good stories.

Back again to Atlanta and then off to Des Moines.

The air journey from Atlanta to Des Moines started as a straightforward, rapid flight but after a couple of hours we were caught in a blizzard and the speed slowed down. I noticed that the wings were getting very loaded with ice and snow. Some of the passengers coming from the warm south did not expect this and were dressed in light summer-clothing. We were delayed over an hour and ultimately arrived at Des Moines on a snow-covered aerodrome. I was taken to the hotel and was indeed glad to have arrived safely. On the following day, a Sunday, I woke early, packed my bags and went downstairs to breakfast after which I returned to my room and lay down on the bed to read the Sunday newspapers. Suddenly the door flew open and a coloured girl rushed in shouting "The hotel is on fire". I picked up my bags and went for the elevator, but it was not working so I started to walk down the stairs. I think I was on the sixth floor. The place was now full of smoke and three or four floors down people were struggling down the crowded stairway, mostly dressed in their night attire. I saw a bell-boy and presuaded him to take my bags. By the time I reached the second floor the firemen with their hoses were coming up the stairs and the ground floor was covered in water. I heard that the fire was two floors above my room and that someone had turned off the electricity supply and that a lift girl had been trapped between two floors. There were no casualties but there was a certain amount of chaos. I took a taxi to Dr. Bierring, the state Health Commissioner, and told him of the lack of organisation of the staff in the emergency and the consequent confusion and I was told that this was the third fire at this hotel in the last few years. I should hate to be in a really big hotel fire after a taste of what it could be like. My wife was in New York and was told of my escape and safety before she had heard of the fire !

I then travelled by train with Dr. Bierring to Iowa City to address the Faculty at the University where the chair was taken by Dr. Robert Harden, now the Dean, who had been attached to the Blood Transfusion Service in Bristol during the war and with whom we had become very friendly.

Then to Cincinnati. This was my first visit to that Mid-West City and, for the first time, I missed companionship, my wife having left me to go via New York to Torronto. On arrival I decided to go in the evening to have a really good dinner somewhere but the hotel manager knew of no better place than his own hotel ! I knew no-one or no place besides so I had to be satisfied. I found the dining room almost empty. The waiter told me there was a big private dinner in another part of the hotel—the occasion being St. Patrick's Day. "But," I said, "I did not know you had many Irish in Cincinnati". "Oh no sir—very few Irish but it is an opportunity for a good and merry dinner !"

I reported to the Consul in the morning and he invited me to tea on the Sunday to meet Miss Colston of Bristol descent with a name well-known in that city. She was a prominent citizen of Cincinnatti and full of good works. We had a pleasant chat—she had visited the city of her ancestors. Trying to be pleasant to her I told her I would tell the City Fathers of Bristol that I had met a descendant of Edward Colston. "No, please, don't," she said. "He was a bachelor !" I shall be more cautious next time.

At Cincinnatti I was taken on the Sunday to join the two who "did" "World Front" on the radio. I was introduced and asked how would I tackle the problem of prostitution. My answer was quite frank and simple. I would have social workers investigate the cause, have them properly analysed and then proceed to treat the cause. That was the only way a Preventive Medicine Man could look at the problem and in the end it was the only sure way of tackling it. Of course the answer was not a good one—time was "inopportune". In the meantime let's go on treating the symptoms ! It was an interesting experience.

Louisville Kentucky was interesting. My first engagement was a lunch with a small party of about a dozen as a guest of the Dean of the Faculty of Medicine. Present also was the Mayor, a jolly and humourous man free from all ostentation. He presented me with the flag and key to the city. I was presented to the author of *The King and I* and her husband. I could not help being reminded of my son's remark one day, "When I settle down in practice I shall look forward to theday when walking the streets people will say—there goes Dr. Martin and his father. I shall then know I've got there !" In my talks about the British Health Services, the one to the doctors was not appreciated by them ; they thought it was propaganda ! As a critic of its weaknesses there was nothing further from my mind.

At St. Louis, the great industrial city in the centre of the United States, there wasmuch to see and my stay there was made especially pleasant by a friendly and happy British Consul who had arranged my time-table. At a large rotary luncheon we started with the Star Spangled Banner and then the Welsh Land of my Fathers. This took me by surprise and I asked the chairman, an Irishman, if there were many Welsh people in the city. He did not know, but the pianist was the director of music for the education service and, as I learned later, was a Welshman. I was presented with a certificate of appreciation for my address. On my way back to the hotel the television was booming out at a bar and I turned in and, by good luck, had a high seat at the bar with a good view. The Kefauver trial of the gangsters was on in Washington and business had slowed down to watch the proceedings on T.V. There was much interest in "Greasy thumb goosy" or something of the kind who had an association with St. Louis. Having emptied my glass the man next to me turned and said "Another ?" I said, "No thanks". He looked again and said "Dr. Parry ?" I said "Yes, how did you know ?" He replied, "I read my papers". I spent most of the following day with a trades union leader who had formed an industrial medical service and was employing three or four full-time doctors. He found it very hard-going against the wishes of the medical profession but he was a stubborn fighter with strong convictions although his health was not good. I spent much of my spare time with the Consul and was entertained at his home by his wife and himself. He was the best type of English public schoolboy, natural, with a keen sense of humour and charm. It was no wonder that he was popular with the Americans and I only wish more of the British people I met had been of the same mould. Our image in the U.S. would have improved accordingly.

I have already referred to my visits to Chicago which had to be passed through to get anywhere by rail. In Detroit I found my programme badly arranged and difficult to fulfil until the Health Commissioner took me in hand. First of all there was a meeting of the Civil Defence Medical Service where the Health Commissioner had prepared an excellent report. When, at the end of the meeting, I was asked for comments from our experience on this side of the ocean I suggested that a good deal of attention could be given to care of the dead to "Maintain the morale of the living". Identification, attendants to care for the bodies and plenty of coffins—we had found these of great importance during the bombing in Bristol. When the evening papers came out much attention was paid, in large headlines, to my remarks. Three medical meetings were being held in different parts of the city that evening and I was rushed to all three and asked to say a few words. Detroit came into my life again in 1956 when I was visiting professor at Yale. I was invited to lecture in Ann Arbor and our friends, Dr. and Mrs. Henry Vaughan, spent the best part of the day taking us through the lovely city and to see the Ford Museum which is indeed worth a visit.

A visit to New Haven, Yale, followed under the guidance of Dr. Ira Hiscock, Chief of the School of Public Health, which I was to have the privilege of serving in 1956 as a visiting professor, and the honour of dining in the home of Professor and Mrs. Winslow. There, also, I met a young English lady who had served a term as a district midwife in Kentucky going about on horseback. She was thrilled with the life.

At Providence, Rhode Island, on a Sunday I addressed two meetings at the lovely home of the Chairman of the English Speaking Union, the second meeting consisting of the Faculty of Browns University. I must have looked tired—and no wonder—because the lady of the house made me lie on a couch under a rug and put on long-playing records of soft music for nearly an hour. I confess it did me a world of good.

I was asked back to John Hopkins, Baltimore, once again to meet my old friends. They took over a club dining-hall for a Saturday evening jollification and it was indeed a memorable occasion. No wonder in the morning when I addressed a civil defence meeting I stressed the importance and value of clean water !

During a visit to Washington we attended a memorable dinner-party at the house of Mr. Morgan, Counsellor at the British Embassy. He really had settled in America and had an estate in California. Originally from Swansea, he had married a sister-in-law of Colonel

Lindbergh and, after her death, had married her sister. In his house in the centre of Washington his dining-room contained a good Welsh dresser and a fine collection of Swansea china. At the dinner party we met the reporter who had dared to criticise the singing of President Truman's daughter and, for his trouble, he had had a letter sharply rebuking him. This he had sold as a valuable historical document! We also heard of the British Government's venture with chickens in Gambia where chickens can't survive! It only cost us four million pounds, or was it eight, and we had not heard of the affair in Britain—I wished I had never heard it. But the Americans knew all about it—were we censored or were we?

My final assignment before leaving was to Pottsville, Pennsylvania, to address a joint meeting of the Welsh Society and the Medical Society after dinner! It was quite a problem but it passed off—neither one thing nor the other.

My host, called Jones, was a wealthy coal-mine owner and before the meeting he had sent me in the charge of his manager to see the workings of a surface mine. It reminded me very much of the way the beautiful South Wales countryside had been spoiled. I asked if they intended to level the slag heaps as they went along but the manager's reply was, "It would not pay". That had a modern British ring about it! After the meeting I went with Mr. Jones in his car from his town-house to his farm twenty miles or so away. It was a big farm divided into parts according to the age of the cattle and their purpose. He had brought his bulldozers in and levelled some of the hillocks to make the land easier to work. He was a most interesting man, capable and far-seeing. The son of a former South Wales miner, he had worked his way, by hard work, to be a wealthy man. He told of his visit to his father's native village in South Wales. He went to the village "pub", his father had mentioned and there met many young miners but none of his father's generation. He stood drinks all round and one youngster said in a loud voice, "Look at that damn Yank throwing his money about". A sensitive man, he left the "pub" and left Wales never to return again. How stupid and inhospitable some people can be! Before I left in the morning he showed me his deep-freeze room of substantial size, something like 16 ft. x 16 ft. and divided into compartments—fish, fruit and meat. His agent in Chicago saw to it that he had carcasses of prime beef at the right time, had it butchered and delivered—the same with the other foodstuffs. It appeared that he supplied the meat and other food for all public dinners, of which he approved, in Pottsville, including the one I attended the night before. He asked me what I would like to take home with me. I had to think hard—hams, joints—no a tin of bully-beef weighing seven pounds, the easiest of all to transport. It was most acceptable in 1951 and of excellent quality.

It is interesting to read now, in 1969, the conclusions I reached after my two "goodwill" tours to the U.S.A. when I was reporting back to Bristol Council after my second visit.

Here is a summary of my impressions :—

"The struggle for existence is keen : the slacker is passed by. But they are very kind to those who fall by the wayside. Their hospitality to the visitor, or at least to me, was unsurpassable. They are blunt in their criticism. Their radio and newspapers give accounts of the exceptions, the murders, the gangsters, the mentally subnormal and these become accepted almost as ' the average ' although they are the exceptions not only for their own country but for other countries as well. And so ordinary people like myself are accepted there because we give the blunt, simple story of our lives as they are—our achievements and our failures. They are intolerant and suspicious of those who are on their dignity and who refuse to acknowledge any faults ; as also they are of those who see nothing right with "the old country". I was deeply impressed with their energy, enthusiasm and conviction and it made me wonder if after all we in this country have not very nearly made a religion of compromise so that our children hardly understand our conception of right and wrong."

CHAPTER VI

FOUR MONTHS IN GREECE WITH THE AMERICAN MISSION, 1949

ONE day in January, 1949, I was called to the telephone to speak to the Deputy Chief M.O. of the Ministry of Health. He wanted to know if I would be interested in going to Greece to advise the American Mission on the medical aspects of their social insurance administration. Of course I was interested ! An application was made by the Ministry through the Town Clerk to release me from my duties as Medical Officer of Health and Professor at the University. I was summoned to meet the full City Council so that the matter might be discussed in my presence. Of course, such a project could not hope to obtain unanimous support but I was surprised to see how little opposition was shown to granting me leave. One fluent alderman wished to know how a "monoglot Englishman" (that's me !) could work with a people whose language was so different. The Lord Mayor turned to me for a reply. "I think, Lord Mayor, that Welsh will be Greek to those people" !—the discussion closed and I was released. I was asked to meet the American chief of that branch of the Mission, Mr. Oscar Powell. We met at the Atheneum in London and seemed to understand each other without any trouble. Ever since then he and his wife have been included amongst our best friends.

My task was to advise the American Mission on the Medical aspects of the social insurance scheme for industrial workers and their families since, as a result of the world war followed by the civil war, the scheme had become bankrupt. There were other aspects which surprised us not a little, such as when the manager of one industrial firm which he had served in that capacity for several years stated that there were dozens of redundant workers still on full pay who never turned up at the works, although on one occasion one had come to complain that he had not had a rise in wages with the other workmen. He had not been to work for fifteen years. It was a difficult task for the Mission to set the old scheme on a sound basis and several first class American administrators had been assigned under Mr. Powell to put it right. They approached the problem with open minds, great skill and generosity. In fact they were underwriting it.

Travelling in Greece was not always easy or comfortable. My Chief, Oscar Powell, was always accompanied by a Greek soldier with a sub-machine gun but we never had much confidence in his knowledge or skill should he have been required to use the weapon. He caused us no end of delay whenever we came to an army post because they accepted our passes but always queried the guard's. All the same he was very tolerant and patient and although we couldn't understand what he said he always sounded most apologetic ! On the occasions when I had to travel some distance to see a hospital I was thoroughly scared by the reckless driving. It appeared, although it was probably not really so, that the drivers accelerated when they saw a pedestrian crossing the road—after, of course, they had blown their horns loud and clear ! In Greece the narrow roads, sharp corners on precipitous drives, of which there were plenty, appeared to make little difference to the speed. Even so, it was always more comfortable on ' terra firma ' than in the air, especially when we heard that the plane following the one by which we travelled from Salonika had blown up in the air.

One of my greatest pleasures was to plan several health centres for general practitioners—one in Heraclion, Crete, one in Volos, one on the Attica peninsula and several in Athens, from which the doctors could provide both treatment and organised preventive services. Sites have already been found and the architects are at work. I hope one day I shall be able to go and see them in operation.

A memorable journey by sea from Patras to Corfu was undertaken because we had been invited to a tea party at the luxurious bungalow which the late King had presented to his Chamberlain in appreciation of his loyalty in difficult times. We found that this tea party had been arranged by the Greek Director of I.K.A. who was a cousin of the Chamberlain and there were two other cousins at the party, one being the Minister of the Navy. We saw an opportunity for that journey which we must take to Corfu and then and there persuaded the Minister to take us. We left Patras at mid-day on a Sunday in a corvette, sailed through the narrows, arrested a few smugglers on the way and arrived in Corfu late in the evening. We finished our tasks and left at midnight, sleeping on deck, to arrive at Patras in daylight. Our Greek interpreter pointed out to us the Rock of Ulysses which we passed on our right as we went to Corfu. The story that made this rock famous tells of twenty young mothers who jumped down with their babies in arms and killed themselves rather than submit when surrounded by the Turks. We also saw Missologlu where Lord Byron, a great hero to the Greeks, died fighting for Greek independence.

Where a country has been occupied by foreigners, be the occupying forces military or civilian, it tends to divide the native people, breeding distrust and suspicion amongst them, for some co-operate with the occupiers and are looked upon as traitors by those who remain loyal to their own country. Many ordinary Greek tradesmen told me quite categorically that the Greeks never trusted each other but I think that was an exaggeration.

In many of the provincial towns hardly any medical services existed and the private doctors struggled against great odds, depending entirely on their own resources. In one such town, Aegion, about twelve to fifteen miles from Patras, a town of 20,000 people, nearly all working-class, they had one hospital of forty beds, which belonged to the local authority but was subject to the control of the Ministry of the Interior. The local authorities are so poor, having hardly any source of income, that they are quite unable to provide the services they would like. In this town the hospital board could not afford to feed the patients so they had to get their relations to bring them their food. There was an X-ray machine still in its packing, presented by U.N.R.A. three years before but no one to work it. The hospital, however, was built with the usual Greek taste for beauty on a lovely site and it could be modernised and staffed properly if the finances were forthcoming. An offer was made by us on behalf of the Institute of Social Insurance to take it over and provide, after extending it, a first-class service, in and out-patient, for all the people of the town. But nothing happened because—same old story—the municipality objected to relinquishing control. Under similar circumstances in another town I regret to say that my own medical colleagues who were doing well out of their private nursing homes, because of lack of reasonable hospital facilities, were fighting tooth and nail against the development of the local hospital by the Institute. On the whole, however, the attitude of the profession was very similar to that of the majority in our country, their chief aim being to help their patients and they did well under difficult circumstances.

There are thousands of children, orphans and refugees, in homes throughout the country, usually being very well-cared for by the Queen's Fund Organisation. There are tens of thousands of refugees in the small provincial towns—just imagine a town the size of Bath having to cope with 15,000—20,000 refugees! In our climate it would be quite impossible, but in Greece the temporary shacks in which these people live in large congested numbers seem to be less harmful to their general health than would be imagined. However, that is only my impression as I was quite unable to find any reliable statistics regarding the people's health. This refugee problem is nothing new to Greece. In 1922, for example, during the war with Turkey, the country found itself saddled with a million and a half additional people, refugees from Asia Minor. They put them in different settlements, usually near the towns, and they are still referrrd to as refugee settlements.

Briefly the scheme we prepared was based on the principle that general practitioners should work from health centres with district nurses and midwives, and that all specialists should have hospital beds, so that the cases which they saw at the dispensary could, if necessary, be admitted to their hospital beds. In addition there was to be direct access to specialists, but very limited and usually through the general practitioner. The idea of doctor-inspector we condemned and insisted that it could be replaced with advantage by an effective system of dealing with complaints by the patients and by a financial check on the prescription through the accounts department.

Malaria used to be extremely prevalent until U.N.R.R.A. took the problem in hand and sprayed the affected parts of the country with D.D.T. This has been followed up by the Americans. It means great expense in trained staff and equipment, including planes, and I hope the Greeks will be able to keep up the good work. Malaria is now very infrequent and many of the doctors have suffered much financially—one wrote a very strong letter to the Mission about the new system which had deprived him of his living. In the old days with his black bag he could earn enough in three months to keep him for the rest of the year.

I saw the disadvantages of democracy in Greece. The so-called representatives of the people tended to stick to their posts at all costs and so hindered progress more often than not. On one occasion my Chief said he had an offer of an X-ray apparatus, at the time worth £4,000 or £5,000, and he sent the offer to the management committee of I.K.A. They were paid for attendance at the committee meetings and they had met there three times before our patience was exhausted. After the first meeting they had written a charming thank-you letter saying they would consider it ; after the second they wanted to know the name of the makers, and after the third meeting they asked if they could choose their own make ! We gave them a limited time to say "this one—yea or nay". Sometimes in this country members of committees are considered to be "good committee" people becasue they have neither conviction nor moral courage to express their own views but are good people otherwise. The idea has gone abroad that it is evil not to compromise. Such persons should be persuaded to write their views in private and then get someone else to read these views out in committee ! Surely there is every reason why the ballot is so important if true democracy is to survive.

Several times I had a pleasant feeling of being proud of my own country and its people. I heard a Greek interpreter at Salonika insisting that the Greek nation has the right to grumble and grouse at us for did we not fight for Greek independence and had we not been Greece's godmother ever since. And again when the scholarly Bishop of Corinth paid a mighty tribute to the late William Temple and to our former Bishop Woodward when I visited him in his home. On another occasion a guerilla fighter who was our driver told us in detail and with great feeling how all but five of the band of New Zealanders died on the beaches of Canea fighting for the British cause. And last, but not least, our guide on the Acropolis, after showing us the gold statue of Athaene and the Temple of Hygeia, took us to a spot and said with pride "There sat Sir Winston Churchill sketching and looking in that direction".

It was these impressions of Greece and my task with the Mission that I passed on to the City Fathers of Bristol when I addressed them soon after my return. I regret that I have had no opportunity to revisit the country again. No doubt many of the problems have been worked out and improvements made in the Health Services in the last twenty years.

The following is an extract from a talk to the Medical students given soon after my return from Greece :

"No doctor brought up in the tradition of British medicine can but be thrilled at the opportunity of visiting Greece, the homeland of Hippocrates. It is very tempting to let my thoughts wander and talk to you about ancient Greece—the remains of the temples of Aesculapius at Epidaurus and on the side of the Acropolis in Athens ; or to describe to you the Aesculapian corner in the museum at Corinth

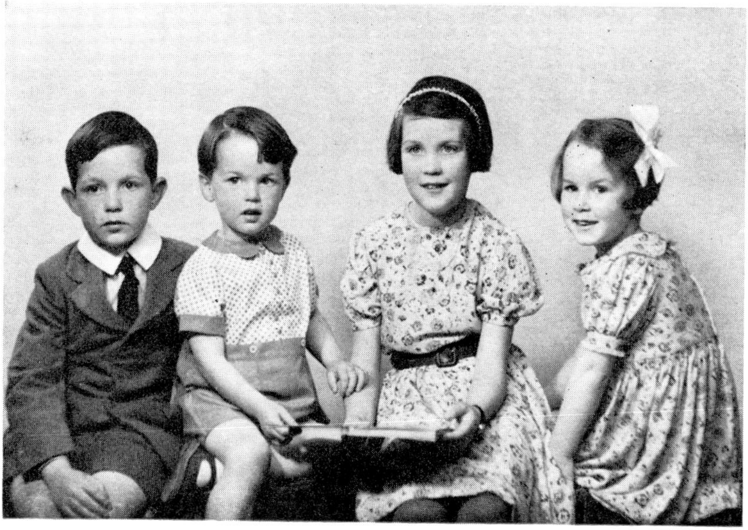

The children before their evacuation to Canada. The original picture was rescued from the rubble after the complete destruction of the Health Office, 40 Prince Street, Bristol in 1940

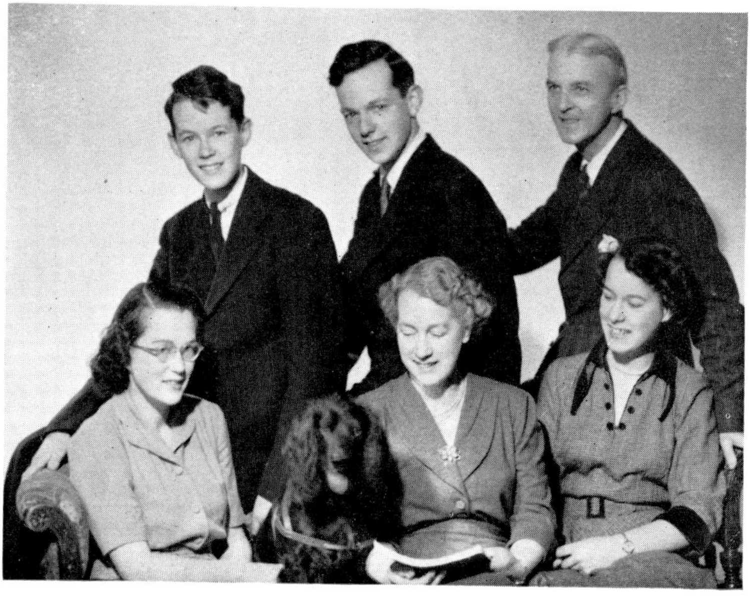

The family reunited after the war

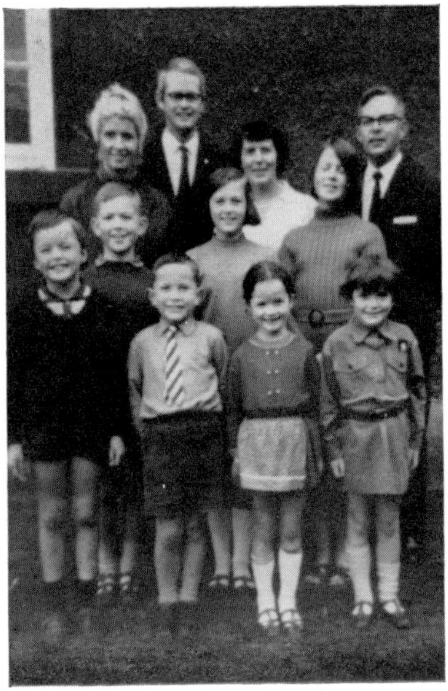

The two sons with their
wives and family, 1969

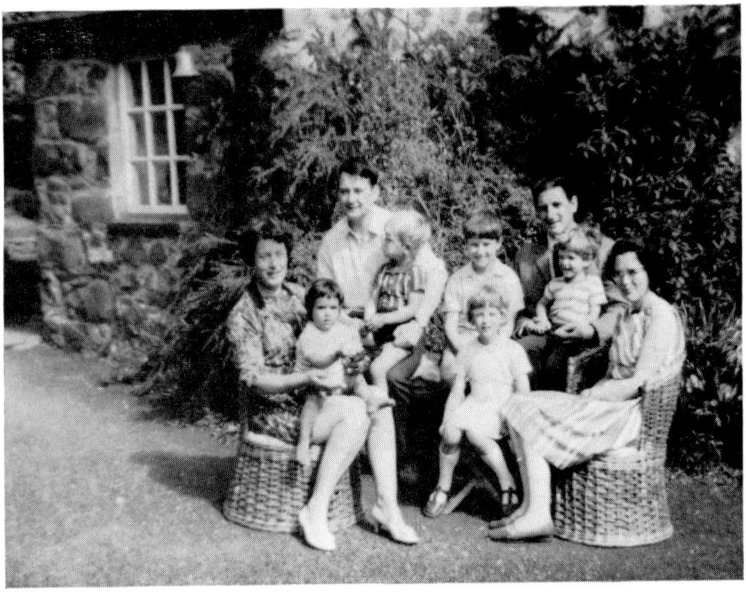

The two daughters with husbands and family (1969)

where there was a collection of ancient medical instruments and small models of parts of the body in pottery, gold or silver. It appears to have been the custom to deposit these models at the Aesculapian shrine after the part had been cured. It does not require a statistician to tell what part of the body was most frequently affected and thereafter cured, although it might be that these particular tokens just signified the gratitude of the patients—some being more grateful than others.

But I cannot pass by without saying a little about these temples of Aesculapius ; after all we did inherit the scientific spirit from the Greeks. It is quite evident from the situation of these temples and their planning that medical practice in them was not all jugglery. The temples in Athens is on the south side of the Acropolis and is protected from the north whence come the cold north winds that come in late winter and early spring—the site is therefore a wonderful suntrap. The Aesculapian consists of a temple and a nearby theatre ; there is a platform for sunbathing and a small running stream that is looked upon as sacred and was no doubt most useful for treatment. We know what can be done with sunshine and water today in the prevention and treatment of disease. The ancient Greeks knew it also in their day when they established the Aesculapeian at Athens about 420 B.C. and most probably it was visited by the great Hippocrates himself. These Aesculapeians were the earliest example of medical centres—a little more elaborate than our present day centres and hospitals and under lay administration which was more justified in those days than today, the auxiliary services hardly required medical skill to organise them."

The Greeks are charming people—stubborn in their views and excitable, but, in their own homes, cultured, artistic and hospitable. They love beautiful things and the florists, whose shops are full of roses, carnations and many other flowers, all seem to make a good living. Their architecture, ancient and modern, is admired the world over. I visited several homes, some of which were newly built, and the planning was good and the workmanship excellent.

There were several incidents during my stay in Greece that impressed themselves most deeply on my memory, and I feel that some of these are worth recording.

It was a lovely Sunday morning and I was sitting in the King George Hotel, which had been taken over by the Americans, and where I had a room. I was talking to an American who had been one of the senior press correspondents on a similar mission to Korea and he was most enlightening on that country and its people of whom I knew nothing. We decided to take a walk and, as usually happened, we found ourselves wending our way towards the Acropolis. On our way we met or joined with many young Greeks—men and women—parading in their Sunday best as was their custom, and we were greatly impressed by their good taste and charm. We wandered towards the entrance of the Acropolis but instead of entering I persuaded him to cross the road and stand where I imagined St. Paul had stood when he made that famous speech to the Greek intelligentsia and business men (see Acts, ch. 17). We stood on the Areopagus and could see, as he could, the whole of the old city, now in ruins, the ruins of the Temple of Zeus down below and, on the right above us, the Acropolis with its ruined temples. Amongst them can be had a glimpse of a smaller temple identified as that to the ' Unknown God '.

I had never felt the full significance of that sermon of St. Paul until I stood with my American friend where St. Paul had stood nearly two thousand years ago. My friend was more aware of modern literature and news, but I was glad to escape to the distant past.

Then there was a visit with a doctor to his native village, and let us not forget that the civil war was still being waged. Through my interpreter he expressed himself as being anxious for me to taste the lemonade made in his village—the best in Greece. We enjoyed the ride immensely and when we reached the village he vanished. Presently he returned with a priest, an old school pal, and glasses of lemonade. It certainly was excellent lemonade. I was told to watch carefully and this I did while the two old friends chatted and joked and slapped each other on the shoulder. Presently the doctor pulled the cloak aside, gripped the wrists of the priest, who in his right hand held a loaded revolver. Then the doctor proclaimed that the priest had been responsible for the death of more communists than anyone else in Greece.

During my stay in Athens there were two unique ceremonial parades the like of which I had never before seen. One of these was the occasion of the funeral of the Archbishop of the Greek Church. His body was borne on a gun-carriage covered in white, his face, with the long, flowing beard, exposed to view. Preceeding the gun-carriage was the King in his Rolls Royce and army chiefs, followed by many celebrities in their Cadillacs. We were fortunate in that my room at the King George Hotel opened onto a verandah overlooking Constitution Square round which the procession passed and so I had a close view of the body and the impressive parade.

We also saw the Easter parade and for a description of this event I am indebted to my wife who was with me during the Easter celebrations.

"I was indeed fortunate to be in Athens at Easter—celebrated by the Greek Orthodox Church one week later than in our country. The most impressive part of the celebrations began on Easter Eve. As soon as the sun has set processions start converging on the centre of Athens, Constitution Square, from all parts of the city. We could watch the one from the Church on the summit of Mount Lycabettus, the moving torches looking like a fiery snake coming down the winding road. One such procession was preceded by soldiers pulling Christ's bier accompanied by a band playing the Dead March. Everyone flocked to the Cathedral with the King and his Ministers. The Archbishop said 'Christ is risen' and held up a lighted candle, and it seemed as though everyone did carry one, and lit theirs in turn from their neighbour's. As soon as the King had passed in his car, still holding his lighted candle, the crowd moved away, each hoping to reach home with his or her candle still burning as that would mean good fortune in the coming year. The cry 'Christ is risen' was heard on all sides with the answer 'He is risen indeed'. We mingled with the crowds and eventually reached our hotel at the end of a very moving and memorable evening."

Another occasion I remember very vividly started when my chief decided to go to Crete. A few planes were flying and we made arrangements for four of us with the interpreter to arrive in Crete and be met by a guide who could speak English. Here I must interrupt my story to repeat what I said have so often in the past that you cannot get to know the people of any country unless you understand their language and their method of expressing themselves. The misunderstanding between different peoples can often be traced to this difficulty. In my native country which has now been occupied so long it is not difficult for people like myself, who have spent so much of our lives in England and understand both points-of-view, to realise that the Welsh are often misunderstood by the monoglot English. So I found when I went to Greece and also in Persia. A young American Jewish graduate mastered both languages in a matter of a few weeks and had a great advantage over some of us. The teaching of different languages in school should be of primary consideration. And now to return to my story. We landed on the beach at Heraclion and were met by the Greek interpreter who spoke excellent English. On our way to the town he stopped and told us this story :—"I was here defending the beaches when the Germans landed by air and sea. We killed many, the New Zealanders were magnificent. I saw less than a dozen of them giving the Maori war cry and charging with their bayonets against overwhelming odds. I am proud to have been with them and to have known them—I escaped to the hills to fight another day". When we had done some of our work we realised that it was Easter week and the Greeks with us could only have a good meal if we were 'bona fide' travellers. So we became just that by going for a long run in our jeeps. On our way back we stopped at a Turkish restaurant on the outskirts of the town of Heraclion. Alas, I had laryngitis and was not feeling too well but I enjoyed the meal very much all the same—choice of delicious meat wrapped in olive leaves and meats from the common dish with rice and sauces followed by the oranges of Crete such as I had never seen before. We were accommodated for the night in a half-tumbled-down house which at one time had been the home of a wealthy city man. The double room which my Chief and I were to share had one bed and another consisting of a mattress on chairs and a chest of drawers. Mr. Powell insisted on tossing for the bed although I warned him that I usually won the toss—and so I did ! I slept well but he remade the other bed on the floor. A couple of days later we were to catch a plane at Canea but it failed to land there. I was worried as I was due to meet my wife and a friend at Athens Airport that afternoon. We waited hopefully and sure enough another plane arrived but it only had accommodation for two passengers so my Chief and I climbed aboard and flew off. We arrived at Athens airport to find my wife and her friend being rescued by the police liaison officer—they had neither the language to explain nor the money to buy themselves out of their dilemma. They were entirely dependent upon my spare dollars as it was 1949 when our poor country was in the hands of Stafford Cripps, the Chancellor of the Exchequer, and in the doldrums with the pound about to be devalued.

I have already alluded to the ancient health centre, and in particular to the one on the side of the Acropolis. One day my wife and her friend, the widow of a doctor in the Indian Medical Service, and I were sitting on the grassy slope just below the Sanctuary of Aescalapius and overlooking a platform where treatment was given by the physicians amongst whom could have been Hippocrates himself. Our friend asked me to bare my arm and, dipping her hand in the stream that gushed from the sacred spring in the Sanctuary, she made the sign of the Serpent on my arm and said "Now you are a *real* physician." An extra to the Hippocratic Oath !

Whilst visiting the British Ambassador in Athens, my wife and I were introduced to a prominent Turkish citizen, an anglophile and a great friend of the Ambassador. We told him that we had high hopes of being able to escape from duty and spend a few days in Istanbul. He gave us a few suggestions on where to stay and told us he would send to our hotel a reliable guide to show us round wherever we wanted to go. Mr. and Mrs. Powell, and my wife and I departed on a Turkish ship from Pireus and sailed for Istanbul through the Dardenelles. It was a very pleasant trip, and as far as I was concerned crammed with historical memories. One amusing incident occurred. There was a Turkish orchestra playing on board during dinner and they played a selection of English and Welsh tunes including "The Ash Grove" and "Men of Harlech". I went to the band leader and tried to tell him how delighted we were that he should honour the only Britishers present by playing a selection of our songs. "Oh" said he, "is that what they are ?" Rather deflating for our pride !

We found our way to an hotel that was reasonably comfortable, although we were told that a luxury hotel on the outskirts was the usual American resort. However, this one suited our pockets better.

The following morning Kemel arrived—this guide we had expected. He spoke English perfectly and we discovered that he had married an English woman from London and had an only daughter who worked in a London bank. He used to visit them at least twice a year taking with him two prayer rugs, one, so he said, especially for Sundays, but returned with neither, thus clearing his expenses. He had been a well-known boxer and described several fights in London against English boxers. He had fought for Turkey in the world war and had been adjutant to Kemel Ataturk during the revolution. He spoke with much respect for that great patriot and always stood to attention when his name was mentioned. He took us to see the many beautiful mosques and round the old city walls, but not the least exciting was our visit to the bazaar and market which had been the Sultan's stables. We would certainly not have felt safe without Kemel's assistance in the crowded alleys and at one moment I had to summon help. I understand this bazaar has since been destroyed by fire.

Our Turkish friend took us to his house on the Bosphorus and there we had tea with his wife and son in their lovely garden overlooking the domes and minarets of Istanbul and the Golden Horn bridge. There was a small pond in the garden and we listened to the strange sound of singing frogs ! He showed us his lovely home and his remaining treasures, for during the last war he had narrowly escaped death at the hands of Hitler's troops in Rumania by escaping from hospital. His wife spoke a little English and French so we were able to communicate fairly well. Their only son had been trained as an engineer in Glasgow where he had been during the war and, of course, he spoke English very well. We were invited by this charming family to join them on a day's cruise in the Sea of Marmora and visit the islands of Principo and the shores of Asia Minor. On disembarking at one of the islands we went for a drive in an open cart with wicker seats, drawn by two horses and covered with a gay canopy. The islands were very hilly and covered with large bushes of Mediterranian Heath and Judas trees, in full bloom. After a delightful Turkish lunch we re-embarked and sailed across to the other side of the Bosphorus where we landed and were taken for an interesting drive along the coast as far as Scutari to see the old hospital where Florence Nightingale looked after the sick and wounded during the Crimean War.

We decided to fly back to Athens on different planes and went to the airport to make arrangements. There I found a Welshman, the son of a South Wales miner, in charge of the B.E.A. office. He had married a Turkish girl. He asked me to take a message back to his widowed mother, and this I tried to do.

When I arrived back in Athens soon after my wife's plane had landed I found her in difficulties with the immigration officials as we had forgotten to obtain a re-entry permit to stay on in Greece. Fortunately I recognised a police liaison officer who knew me and he was able to intervene and my wife was allowed to stay.

A couple of weeks later my wife decided to fly back home. Passing the customs in front of her was a man with side-whiskers, a deerstalking hat and plus-fours and smoking a Peterson pipe. I tapped him on the shoulder and said "Oxford or Cambridge ?" "Cambridge" said he without looking up. "What College ?" "Queens," again without turning round. "For the sake of my great, great, great uncle, will you keep an eye on my wife ? She is coming to London with you". He suddenly turned round and said, "Who was your great, great, great uncle ?" "His name was David Hughes." "Good heavens, he was one of the Founders of our library and I am the Librarian." I understand that sleep overtook the travellers—maybe that is the best way to pass the hours !

I stayed another month to finish my task.

CHAPTER VII

SOME VISITORS TO BRISTOL, 1930—1956

During our nearly thirty years in Bristol we had the privilege of acting as hosts to many interesting people. Sometimes they stayed with us for a night or two, but sometimes it was a hasty visit when we had to make the most of their company.

The first name that occurs to me is Andrija Stampar—it was about 1937—who was then Chief Medical Officer to Yugoslavia. He spent several days with me visiting different branches of the health and hospital services. It was his reaction to what he saw, his comments and suggestions, and particularly his accounts of visits to other countries as well as a vivid description of his own country, that interested us most. He had spent the best part of three years in China studying the public health in some of the provinces. His report to the League of Nations, published by them in their reports are classics on the subject and well worth reading today. One evening by the fire he described the problems in his own country where the King had been assasinated. "What did he expect ?" he said, "Who rules by the sword must die by the sword."

The problems of Yugoslavia were mainly due to the fact that the country was not united. There were five different groups of people whose customs, religion and points-of-view on social life differed. There were the politicians, the officials of local and central government, the police and the army. They all had their "interests". "I envy you," he said, "your opportunity in this city. I don't think much of your buildings, they are a little mean, don't you think ? But I suppose you couldn't help it. But the people and their representatives think they have done it all—they use the facilities and respect them. It's very different in our country—the people wouldn't trust the officials, and however wonderful our buildings or our services might be, they would not use them."

I would like to know how things stand since the war—I can imagine that the Great War had changed all this under the great leadership of Marshall Tito—who was not even mentioned when we knew Stampar. It was time to retire to bed. I made a final remark—"I just cannot understand you people and why you cannot get on with one another !

Of course, we are five different peoples in this country." "How's that ? I make four." "Well, there are the English, the Scots, the Welsh, the Irish and the Bristolians. I belong to the ancient Welsh people who were driven by force to the mountains of Wales in order to survive. Some, like myself, have ' sneaked ' back to make a living." "Ah ! I see you are one of the Aboriginals." He was a huge, hearty man who enjoyed his food, his sleep and a good joke. In the morning, "Good morning, You Aboriginals know how to make yourselves comfortable !" (We had put a hot water bottle in his bed !)

Dr. Jameson, later Sir Wilson Jameson, told of how Stampar met his first wife. I repeat this only to show that he was a man of quick decision who knew his own mind. He had no use for young women and hardly noticed them. However, one day his sister brought a girl friend to the house. He noticed her, went up to her and said, "What's your name ?" "Mary." "Will you marry me ?" "Yes."—and I am sure she never regretted it. I saw him once more—he was then very famous—as the First President of the World Health Organisation, and the holder of many honours in many countries. I was delighted to be able to acquire, through the American Public Health Association, a copy of his *Selected Papers* recently published. Much of the story I have told you will be found better told in that book. He did me the honour of sending his assistant, Dr Branlio Crzetanovic, a Croat, at Zagret University, to see me—a flying visit only.

Dr. Branlio cleared up one mystery for us. He said there was no such a person as a Yugoslav—they were just Slavs, Croats and so on living together in Yugoslavia. He told me that President Tito and Dr. Stampar lunched together very often, and he invited me to join them. A great oppotrunity missed, alas !

Then there was Dr. Novokowski, in 1938, who was Professor of Public Health at Vilna University. He threw much light for us on the problems of Poland—that poor country which has suffered so much from having powerful, bad neighbours. Such can always be a menace to the peaceful home. He summarised this by saying, "The Russian people are charming people, but their leaders have always been dreadful, and their theories about living are abominable." This was before the last war. I wonder what has happened to him ?

We enjoyed the company of Professor Charles Edward Smith of San Francisco. He was sent by the Rockefeller Foundation on a tour. At that time, before the war, he was a young man and most enthusiastic for the development of public health. He also passed on, having left a fine record behind him.

* * *

Professor W. W. Jameson was external examiner in Public Health at Bristol for three years, and we both looked forward to the week-end golf at Burnham when examination was over. For two office-workers a round of golf in the morning restored our appetites and our good humour. Another in the afternoon assured us of a good night's sleep. We had many serious discussions about the future organisation of the medical services, and we disagreed widely on certain principles. For example, he maintained that centralisation was the only way to crush competition and get real efficiency and in that respect he was a close follower of Edwin Chadwick. I maintained the exact opposite, and I still sincerely believe in decentralisation. It is the only way to get everyone interested in government, and so to get a united people. I argued that the stability of this country rested on strong local government. Besides, standardisation of people and systems never stimulated progress—rather the opposite. From bitter experience I have found that often no approval could be given to schemes by the central government department because it would "set a precedent." If you argued vigorously for your case and there was no reasonable reply then you were accused of being "emotional". How true today also ! Nevertheless we were very good friends to the last. He was a cautious, conventional person with sound common-sense, such as would be expected from Scotland. Aneurin Bevan, a volatile Celt, said to me once "He is the wisest man I have ever met." He must have been a blessing to him in his job as Minister of Health.

* * *

Alexander MacGregor, Medical Officer of Health for Glasgow, was a particularly good friend. We saw a good deal of each other, and we talked much. On most subjects our views coincided, but there was one subject on which we differed vigourosly and I am inclined to think that I ultimately persuaded him to change his mind. It was on the place of multi-storied flats in the housing of the working-class families. I condemned them without mercy where young children were concerned. He had been brought up in such a flat. There are so many arguments one way and the other that there is no place in this book to go into it further. MacGregor was much more of the Celt than the stolid Jameson.

* * *

John Ryle, Regius Professor of Medicine at Cambridge, was a charming man but I did not find him easy to know, although we often met at meetings of the Nuffield Medicine Advisory Council and he stayed with us in our home. He was an authority on gastric and cardiac conditions and his writing on these are classics. A sound thinker and never afraid of new ideas, he was always interesting. He died of heart disease.

* * *

I found Sir Farquar Buzzard, who was the Chairman of the Nuffield Medical Advisory Council, a much more approachable person. He visited Bristol on several occasions and I well remember his advice to me, based upon his personal experience, "Make full notes on everything as it occurs to you." Alas, I did not take his advice.

* * *

I remember walking down past the University one morning after lecturing and Carey Coombs, the famous heart specialist, was standing on the steps. I called on him to join me in the walk. He came down the steps and said he was not feeling too well but he did want to talk to me. Arm-in-arm we walked slowly down. He then told me that at a meeting of the Medical Committee of his hospital the previous evening some of his colleagues had attacked him for developing a small hospital at Winford for heart diseases in children and they accused him of developing it for selfish motives. I knew Cary Coombs well enough to know that it was not true, but I could see that this attack, which had kept him awake all night, had affected him physically. I knew he was sincere in his declaration that he was the only specialist in Bristol, at that time, who depended entirely on his consultant practice without indulging in private practice. When we reached the bottom of Park Street he collapsed. He was a heavy man and I had difficulty in holding him up and dragging him to a shop door. A passer-by called a taxi and I took him to his own hospital. Two weeks later he wrote me a charming letter declaring his gratitude to me, in his first letter after the attack. The cardiac condition from which he was suffering was the one in which he was one of the world's greatest experts. Said he, "I have never known a case recover—I must be the exception which proves the rule." He died the same day, a couple of hours after writing the letter.

* * *

Strangely enough I had a somewhat similar experience with the other outstanding consultant—Hey Groves, the Orthopaedic Surgeon. He turned up in my office one morning and asked to speak to me in private. He then told me this story.

A few evenings before, he had spoken, with his junior assistant, to the Association of Insurance to try to persuade them to help establish an accident fracture department at the teaching hospital. Later at a meeting of the Medical Board of the hospital it was decided to report the two surgeons to the General Medical Council for advertising. "I am on the point of retiring and I cannot face such publicity," he said.

My first reaction was to laugh outright. Here was an unimportant Medical Committee reporting a great surgeon for advertising ! On the B.M.A. world tour with him I had seen him being fetched in Chicago to demonstrate his own operation on the ankle. In Australia he had been honoured with an Honorary Fellowship ; yet now his own colleagues were reporting him to the General Medical Council for 'advertising'—when, in fact, he was appealing for funds to develop the voluntary hospital.

"What shall I do ?"

"You are the Vice-President of the Royal College of Surgeons. When is your next meeting ?"

"This week."

"Then speak to your President" (Sir Alfred, later Lord Webb Johnson), "and tell him the story you have told me. He was my chief at the Middlesex Hospital. Blame me for troubling him."

Ten days later Hey Groves reported back to me. He had followed my suggestion. It so happened they were appointing their representative on the General Medical Council, and it was decided to appoint the Vice President, Mr. Hey Groves ! !

* * *

Dr. Walter Bierring, State Health Commissioner for Iowa, was a most interesting person. I have a photograph of him before me now. I first met him in New York at a meeting of the American Public Health Association in 1943. He had an artificial leg, having lost his own as a boy when he fell off a train in the Middle-West while selling newspapers. It was then that he became more determined than ever to become a doctor and when he died, well in his eighties, he had been a Professor of Pathology for twenty years, a Professor of Medicine for twenty years and he was completing his twentieth year in public health as Health Commissioner for Iowa. I have never heard of that record equalled, much less beaten.

In 1953, a few years before he died he decided once again to visit his old haunts in Europe, and he stayed in Bristol for a few days. He was of Danish extraction and had studied in Paris under the great Louis Pasteur, and still had the notes he had taken at his lectures. He was a personal friend of William Osler, and he spent several days at Oxford looking for ' memorials ' of the great doctor. I saw him in 1951, when I went by air from Atlanta to Iowa.

★ ★ ★

There were amusing days during the "phoney war" when Bristol was considered "a safe city". Important departments were evacuated to the city, including the B.B.C. I, as a senior field officer, was made the field evacuation officer. But they forgot to give me "the code", and when "secretive looking agents" came along and said, "We are L.O.P.", or some other strange letters sometimes with numbers, I had to look wise and send the Health Inspector with them to find their allocation.

Tommy Handley descended upon us amongst others. Shall we ever forget his programmes, and how we enjoyed them !

Bristol later on had some five hundred or more air-raids, with casualties of fifteen hundred killed and many times more wounded. Two thirds of the houses were damaged or destroyed. My figures are from memory and I have no wish to verify them. Let us not be reminded of those dreadful days.

★ ★ ★

Dr. Charles Best and Dr. Llew Little came to see us in 1943 when they were over from Canada discussing with experts in this country a cure for sea-sickness. After a dinner at the Mansion House with the Lord Mayor we spent a very happy evening together. They described their experience researching with Dr. Banting when they discovered insulin. No doubt that story can be better and more accurately told by others, but I hope I may be forgiven if I repeat one account he gave us of the many applications made to them for some insulin to save a life. He had to refuse because insufficient material was at hand for research for them to part with any at that stage. That application came from Dean Inge, the famous "gloomy Dean" of St. Paul's. His daughter was dying of diabetes but they replied to him as they did to all the others. He wrote back that under the circumstances he must not and could not expect any insulin. The girl died and now the gloomy Dean, too, is dead. "The good is oft interred with their bones."

* * *

In May 1946 Dr. Wals Von Greyerz, Commissioner for the Hospitals of Stockholm, came over and spent a little while with us. His description of Sweden during the war was of great interest. The sympathy of most of the Swedes was definitely with the Norwegians but they could do very little for them. However, they did form "an underground army" to save as many as possible of the young Norwegians who were forced to escape from the enemy. His vivid description of his wife's illness and death and his distress was heart-rending. After this had happened he went out skiing alone in the mountains to try and forget but he failed to take his bearings and was completely lost. Soon he became tired and all he could think about was that he must keep going because if he once stopped he would succumb to sleep and be frozen to death. He had no idea how long this lasted but ultimately he was picked up by a party just as he was giving in. He was a strong built man and he must have put up a great fight but I understand he died some years ago.

In November 1959 a doctor with a long name and a tiny, charming wife (he was a big man), came to spend a couple of days with us. He was the personal doctor of the Prime Minister of Indonesia and had accompanied his chief as far as London, whilst the latter went on to discuss peace problems with the Dutch Government. He was very depressed about the state of his country, and was very bitter about the Dutch, who, he declared, had only come to Indonesia to make their fortunes, and do very little for the people in return. It was possible to sense much trouble in store if he was an example of the "enlightened" Indonesians. He was very fond of flying and I understand he was killed in a flying accident soon afterwards. He was a very fluent speaker in English.

* * *

In February 1950 Dr. Keh-Hung-Li of the Medical College of Peking, China, came and spent a few days in Bristol to see the health services having been sent by the United Nations on a travelling fellowship. He was a small man, obviously very intelligent and quick at picking up points of interest. He spoke English well, and as he said at dinner with our young family who had by now returned from Canada, he was supposed to be a Christian. He devoted much of his talk to the sayings of Confucius of whose wisdom he was a sincere admirer. After a very pleasant evening my eldest son could not understand such an intelligent and charming man being a Communist, so he asked him bluntly. "Are you a Communist?" He hesitated, nodded and said, "I am Chinese."

His comment on the health services of Bristol disturbed me very much. He admired the work we were doing to save the lives of women and children, and our welfare-foods and other services. But he said, "What is the use of our trying to save children's lives for them to die of starvation in the prime of life or even earlier? We have four hundred, maybe five hundred million people in our country—at least two hundred million more than we want. Besides, we have no milk in the large towns in China, only soya bean milk."

Obviously life was expendable in China. I have sent him a Christmas card several times but received no acknowledgment—except a parcel of books from China, on the bacteriological warfare by the Americans. Those must have come from him although there was no note with them. I glanced through them and really he was unjust to my intelligence if he thought that I, who have had a certain amount of scientific training, could possibly believe that evidence. There is a picture of the "Red Dean" looking at the "material". He left, as a memento, a brass incense bowl of the Ming dynasty which I still possess.

* * *

In 1951 a district Commissioner from Burma and his wife, a social worker, both Burmese, spent a few days with us. They werea charming couple and we spent a pleasant evening being enlightened about the conditions in Burma. At least, we realised, the British in Burma had not left behind the bitterness which we had noted when other countries were given their independence. A Lebanese friend explained to us the position in the Lebanon—a very much occupied country. Under the Turks they were allowed to do very much what they liked even to choosing their own Governor. But they were warned, "If you fail to pay your taxes we shall hang your Governor."

The French, on the other hand, tried their best to thrust their language and their culture upon the people to the disadvantage of their own, but in other respects they were more considerate to the people. However, the Lebanese today resent the French occupation more than they do the Turks.

I think there is a lesson for us here in our British countries. I am not a politician but the lesson is there for all to note ! My personal experience during my service with the American mission to Greece in 1949 and in Iran with the World Health Organisation in 1959 was along the same lines. I had the feeling that the leaders of medical thought in these countries did not want to be taught by experts from "young" countries. Did not Greece have Pericles and was not their country the last word in "progress" as far as knowledge, including medicine, and culture were concerned back to the day of Hippocrates ? The same with Persia, the home of Cyrus and Darius and of pioneer doctors long before British and American doctors had been heard of. Who did we think we were to come and throw our weight about ? I had this in mind before I went and maybe that is why my reports and schemes in both countries were accepted and, partly, put into operation, not, of course, as "our" schemes but following our "suggestions."

* * *

In January 1955 a senior Medical Officer from Chile paid us a visit. I am not certain whether or not he was the Chief State Medical Officer. He was most impressed by our cheerfulness. After all the bombardment we had had, and it was very visible in Bristol in 1955, and the long war with its deprivations, we had still kept our chins up. In Chile there was poverty but there had been no war and yet the people were miserable. They went into the shop and found the price of food items was going or had gone up. They could not complain. They just mumbled and paid up, accepting all their trouble as if at the hand of fate, and making no effort to counter it. I do hope we are not going in that direction ourselves in this country ! He saw us soon after the war when the "glorious end of the war" was only just over and our feelings of relief had not arrived at disillusionment. The authorities in Chile, the doctor said, had to overcome not only poverty but also misery, which was a much more difficult task.

* * *

Two most interesting visitors came from Israel and we certainly had a stereoscopic view of the problems this old country and new state had to face, and indeed, was facing very bravely. In 1952 the Medical Officer of Health of Jerusalem came to see the health services of Bristol, and we spent a good deal of time together discussing the different aspects of public health. He was an interesting man, in practice as a surgeon until he was approached by the Prime Minister to take charge of the administration of public health in the city. He was most reluctant to do so but considered it his duty. His was the difficult task of integrating Jews with different backgrounds from the different countries. In fact, the only common denominator was that they called themselves Jews and worshipped accordingly, but in different sects, of which there are several. On leaving he exclaimed, "How different you British people are in your own country from those whom we have met in our country !" I wonder.

The following year the Arab Lady Medical Officer of Health of part of Jerusalem and of the adjacent refugee population spent a few days with us. She was a charming lady, married to a lawyer, and had children of her own. They had had to leave their lovely house in Jerusalem and were now living just outside whence they could see their own home which was now used as a museum. No compensation had been paid. She was very sad that so little had been done to rehabilitate the refugees who seemed to be pawns in a political game but what can any one say ? The position remains unchanged fifteen years later and the Great Powers look on helplessly. One interesting incident occurred when she came over to our house to dinner. My younger daughter said grace, and when she had finished I turned to our guest and asked her :

"What is your religion ?" The reply served me right for my careless lapse.

"Of course, I am a Christian. Christianity, you know, started in my country !"

"Yes, Father. Did you think it had started in Wales?" This from my daughter.

All the same it is a good thing to know a person's religion, for it "gives a line" on his background, and helps towards an appreciation of his points-of-view.

CHAPTER VIII

RETIREMENT

VISITING PROFESSOR TO YALE, 1956

HIGH SHERIFF OF CAERNARVONSHIRE, 1958

I MUST confess that by the time 1955 had arrived I was looking forward to the moment when I could retire. Alas, I had never thought that it would ever come to that pass. But at the beginning of the winter of 1955 I went to the Town Clerk and said I wanted to retire at the earliest possible moment and I gave him six months notice.

A week or two after I had proferred my resignation Dr. Ira Hiscock, Dean of the Public Health School at Yale University, came to visit Bristol. He had been appointed President of the American Public Health Association and asked if during his year of office I would go to Yale as a visiting Professor to help him with his work. I wanted a change and this opportunity suited me admirably. So back I went to the Town Clerk to change my six months notice to three months and at the beginning of 1956 I sailed to the United States for the fourth time on another new adventure.

The City Council gave me an opportunity to say goodbye in full council, and both the Health and Education Medical Services committees gave me farewell meetings.

The City Council decided to ask me to help select my successor. This, however, was a joint appointment with the University and this decision of the Council's was not in accordance with University custom. However, the City Council prevailed. They appointed Dr. Robert Wofinden, my Deputy, to succeed me and they certainly made no mistake. I felt happy to leave a service to which I had devoted my energies for more than a quarter of a century in his able hands.

In my farewell talk at the University party I commended my experience to them—one foot in the Medical Board and of the University and the other in the Health Committee, one foot in the Senate and the other in the City Council but, above all, one foot in the Senior Common Room and the other in the Bristol Club !

1956 saw me installed as visiting Professor at Yale, and it was a most interesting experience. I soon made myself at home and formed many new friendships. I was particularly interested in the University of Yale because of it's association with Wales, and the fact that some of my friends and some of my patients when I practised in North Wales were members of the Yale family. The University started its life as a library which remains its central feature to this day. It was established in New Haven, Connecticut, in 1718 and Governor Elihu Yale, after whom the University was named, made "important gifts of books to the library". Many much greater and more valuable contributions in money and kind have been made since that time by other well-known names in the University's history but the greatness of Elihu Yale's contribution was in its timeliness and his encouragement and his name.

I was extremely interested in the School of Theology, the plan for which had been prepared by Thomas Jefferson for another place but permission had been obtained to use the same for Yale. Thomas Jefferson, the revolutionary, was the great brain of independence days when America declared "U.D.I." from Britain. His was a name much revered in Wales because his mother was Welsh and he is said to have spoken the language of his mother.

No mention of Yale would be complete without a reference to Mory's club, restaurant, pub, or what-you-will. It was my privilege to dine there several times and to get my wife admitted on one special occasion into the sanctum sancotrum. The Wiffenpoofs, that famous Yale choir, exercised their lungs in Mory's and were always appreciated and encouraged by those present.

The centre of New Haven itself has many reminders of colonial days such as the churches of different denominations built on land on the side of the large space in the centre of the town which was apportioned to religious denominations. Other reminders were old colonnial homes which were still occupied but surrounded in many cases by modern development.

I joined the Public Health Faculty at the beginning of the second term and so missed much of the undergraduate teaching, but the post-graduate teaching was in full swing. As far as I can remember the class numbered about thirty and came from different parts of the world—Korea, Vietnam, Iraq and Iran as well as European countries. All the members of the class were working for the degree of Master of

Public Health and were from different branches of Public Health Departments.

The scope of teaching was very much in line with ours in Britain but as there are far more voluntary organisations involved in providing services in U.S.A. their activities had to be reorganised. I found that some of the problems considered were new to me at that time. Alcoholism and drugs had not taken such a hold on this country as they had in the United States, or at least we were not aware of their presence.

I learned much from the Faculty discussion arranged from time to time and one feature of the course is worth recording. For this purpose the class was divided into groups of five to seven students and they were expected to make a study of an approved subject such as "the problem of alcoholism or drugs in the U.S.A." Each group gave an exposition for an hour or more on their subject before the other students and staff at a meeting which we were all expected to attend and to take part in a following discussion. The subject was approved early in the academic year and the exposition took place well on in the third term. You can imagine my surprise when this excellent scheme became the subject of adverse criticism at a Faculty meeting because it was considered "a cause of great strain upon the students" and was it really justified ? I was invited to join in the discussion and found that I felt very critical of the critics. My argument was that these were post-graduate students who would take an active part in health education when they had completed their course. Of course, I argued, it was a strain—the sort of strain to which we should all be subjected before we addressed any meeting if we had prepared our subject properly. I quoted Mr. Arthur Balfour, later Lord Balfour, who declared that he never addressed the House of Commons without feeling nervous. That feeling of tension gives us that extra dose of adrenalin which makes us give of our best. I am glad the scheme was not abandoned and I would like to see it more often adopted in our own universities.

Maybe I brought too much sentiment to bear when discussing the after-effects of disease. This I attribute to my home influences when my father was a Guardian of the Poor. I had heard much about and seen the depressing effect of poverty and its association with disease. I remember making, as usual, a twenty minutes contribution to a class after an excellent lecture on "physical disabilities and how they should be dealt with" by one of the lecturers. My contribution consisted of questions, leaving the answers to be worked out by the listeners. I took as an example infantile paralysis, which had not then been conquered by vaccination. When a baby becomes paralysed what does it mean to the baby ? What does it mean to the mother and father ? What does it mean to the home and what to the local community and the State ? And so through the different stages of life. This is true social medicine and the health officer must bear all these questions in mind.

When I returned from New Haven I came to Criccieth, to the old farmhouse that we had bought a few years earlier and where we hoped to spend the rest of our days. It had been very neglected for some years and my wife had spent most of the time while I had been in Yale making the old house more comfortable.

Soon after my return I was "pricked" as High Sheriff for my home County of Caernarvon and took up my duties in 1958. My first duty was to fetch the Judge of the Assizes from his lodgings in a Rolls Royce, at my expense, and take him to Church through a guard of honour of police. The church service was good because the chaplain spoke well and the police sergeant could sing ! After the service we went to the court, again through a police guard of honour. Here I sat at the Judge's right hand and listened to the proceedings. This happened three times during my term of office and I was fortunate in meeting three of the Queen's Bench Judges who were both human and amusing—out of court. I was told that one of my duties would be to be present at any execution that might follow a court case. Such an event was certain to give me an attack of migrane, though I have never suffered from such a complaint, which could be certified by my doctor wife and excuse me from attending such a spectacle ! In any case I had a fine deputy who could carry out all the duties of the office and, knowing nothing about the job, I felt as efficient as a Minister of the Crown !

It so happened that the Commonwealth Games were being held in Wales that year and some of the water events were held on Lake Padarn, Llanberis, and we had V.I.P. seats for these sports. There were other functions the High Sheriff was dutifully expected to attend and one I especially enjoyed. This was the opening of the New Conway Bridge. An uncle of my great grandfather, called Griffith Davies, a Fellow of the Royal Society and a founder of the Society of Actuaries, was a great mathematician and had advised foreign governments as well as our own Life Assurance Companies. It is said that he was responsible for the calculations that helped the great Telford when planning the Menai Bridge and other undertakings. I could find no definite evidence of his association with the Conway Bridge but I took it for granted and wondered !

To me the honour of being High Sheriff gave me an opportunity as I was settling down to retirement in the county of once more meeting old friends of my early life. In other respects it was time and money wasted and was in fact a somewhat expensive way of getting a good seat at public functions during the year !

I certainly gained a little more information about "the law". Our old Dean of Medicine in Bristol always referred to the law as an ass and this year of apprenticeship convinced me that there was a need in this country for "justice" to replace "law". The rule of law is dominant with us and recognised so throughout the world but reform to bring law into line with justice is of paramount importance. Here is an example of what I mean from a medical angle. It was obvious to a medical man that some of the cases at the Assizes that involved sex crimes could have been avoided if a physical examination had been made by a good physician or surgeon beforehand and treatment been given. To punish the offender and let him loose to commit another offence later is just stupid. But I understand that the judge can do nothing about this. It reminds me of my early days with the school medical service when young children were classified as mentally retarded because they were deaf or partially deaf and were living in a world of their own without hearing what the teacher was saying. In the same way the naughty, inattentive child sometimes had defective eyesight and could not see the blackboard and was punished for his naughtiness when he had only been doing something to occupy his energies. Later on he really became naughty, or in modern parlance, "malajusted".

As a result of my observance of the working of the Court I would go as far as to insist that, where a medical assessor to a judge thinks it necessary, every person before the Assize Court should be physically examined and should never be referred to a psychiatrist before he has been examined and treated for physical disease.

The special lunches were another feature of the High Sheriff's official duties. These were for members of the Bar, officials and friends and took place during the Assizes. My wife took pleasure in choosing the menu and I in selecting the speakers—those who knew least about me but could suggest fluently wat a wonderful fellow I was! I can quite understand why many public personalities like retiring from one job to take up another. We discover when getting a send-off that we have few shortcomings and many qualities and abilities which we had not suspected we possessed and this is so good for our ego, especially when we are wondering if indeed we have done everything possible to make a success of our lives.

There was just one more interesting episode that occurred when I had to attend the Quarter Sessions in my official capacity. My brother was Chairman and in the formal dress of High Sheriff I presented him with "The Precepts". This document is the authority to call the jurors who had been duly summoned, the return having been endorsed with the seal of the High Sheriff.

CHAPTER IX

IRAN FOR THE WORLD HEALTH ORGANISATION, 1959

During the second half of the year when I was High Sheriff I received a communication from the office of the World Health Organisation in Geneva asking if I would be interested in an assignment to Iran to help establish a Higher Institute for Public Health in that country. This appealed to me immensely but I wanted much more information before accepting the offer. I had no idea what the climate was like and I had been warned to keep out of too hot a clime. This problem was soon resolved because we heard that a young Iranian teacher from that country was attending a course of teaching practice in Portmadoc to see how English was being taught as a second language to Welsh-speaking children. We asked her to tea with us and had a long talk about her country including its climate. From all that she told us I became very keen to visit Iran and she persuaded the family that my health would not suffer. She was a Bahai, a religion of which I was ignorant at that time, but I learned more about this and other sects during my stay in Iran. After considering all the information on the subject I decided to try and persuade them that the best course would be for me to visit Iran for three months and study the problem on the spot before writing a report. The official terms of my assignment were "To report on the teaching of Preventive and Social Medicine and the training of Public Health staff in Iran having regard to the establishment of a special Institute for that purpose."

I succeeded in delaying my assignment until I had completed my term as High Sheriff but I was anxious to get to Iran before the hot weather in order to see as much of the country as possible without undue strain.

By the end of April the terms of my appointment had been agreed and I was eager to start my enquiries. There now remained my official appointment as consultant and instructions where and when to report. I waited, then, impatiently, I sent a reply paid cable to the Geneva office. No reply came but a few days later a letter arrived with the official appointment and giving full details. When I reached Geneva I enquired at the office about the reply-paid cable. They produced it. It had been sent to North Wales Pennsylvania, U.S.A.—

a place I had never heard of and, what was most hurtful, it was marked 'not known'! This year, 1969, during a brief holiday in Madeira we met a man who lived in North Wales, Pennsylvania—which proved to us that it does exist!

I spent a week interviewing the heads of the different departments of W.H.O. at the Palais des Nations to get their points-of-view regarding my task and this was most interesting. Amongst them was a doctor who had been a Professor-Director of the Institute of Malariology in Teheran.

From Geneva I went to Cairo and thence to Alexandria to report to the Regional Director of W.H.O. for the Eastern Mediterreanean. He was a Persian and his deputy was Egyptian who had held high office in the Egyptian Medical Service. He had enlightened and progressive views on the subject of public health and had done much to develop rural centres in Egypt. The chief of my particular section was a German and his deputy was Finnish—a truly international group and I cannot speak too highly of their courtesy and their efforts to help me in every way. Socially they were most hospitable. I dined with the Egyptian Deputy-Director and his charming wife in their own home and we discussed the development of public health in Egypt. I attended a violin quartette concert at the home of the German chief of the Education Service station and his wife played the piano. This was a memorable evening. A week went by and I was then ready to travel to Iran.

The first part of the journey, of course, was to Cairo in one of those small planes in which, as a passenger, no-one ever feels very safe. Cairo airport was a most unpleasant place in which to wait and invariably there was a long wait—on one occasion as long as four to five hours. The airport had not been repaired since the British invasion and, as was so often the case in that part of the world, there were too many flies. I understand that all these defects have been repaired more or less since I was there. Then I travelled to Beirut where I had to stay the night and I was booked to stay at the Bristol Hotel which was very modern and expensive. There I saw a B.O.A.C. pilot reading the *Times* of the same day so I went up to ask for the news and we had dinner together. I have considerable sympathy for these officers who find themselves stranded alone usually in a first-class hotel waiting for the time of their departure. Like this pilot they would much rather have been home with their wives and families, sweating in the garden and going to bed on a boiled egg. They would have sacrificed much for this privilege.

It was Ramadan and I realised it was going to be difficult to travel in any Moslem country during this period. I took the Middle East Airways 'bus to the airport and ultimately got on my way to Baghdad and thence to Teheran. It was interesting to watch the shape and contour of the land we passed over and its division into cultivated plots. There was a revolution in Iraq and I felt sorry for the many young men who left the plane at the Baghdad airport. There was a little sound of gunfire which we might not have noticed had we not been told of the revolution. I stayed in the plane although we all had to get out for a few minutes whilst the cabin was sprayed. Whilst waiting I went for a chat to a silent man, an obvious Britisher, and found him to be a Queen's Messenger living in Istanbul and going to Teheran. He was doing this extra job to augment his income—his wife and daughter lived in England.

At Teheran airport with its fine and modern buildings I became thoroughly lost. I was supposed to be met by a United Nations agent but I could find no one remotely resembling such a person. I was on the point of handing myself over to a taxi driver when some one came up and asked me "Are you Mr. X . . . ?" I said "No, but I am glad to hear a word I understand—can you help me ?" He was not in the least inclined to do so but the elderly gentleman whose chauffeur he was heard me and came to the rescue. I explained my predicament and he at once volunteered to take me in his car to a good hotel. He had had much to do with the English when British Petroleum was of some importance in Iran.

The new hotel into which I was installed did not appeal to me either in cleanliness or in the quality of the food and when I was eventually found by Mr. Frank Pauls from Alaska, a laboratory expert with W.H.O., the following morning, he agreed to take me to another hotel nearer the centre of Teheran. Here I had a delightful room looking out on the straight road to Shimran with the grounds of the American Embassy across the road and the snowclad Eburh mountains rising to 12,000 ft. or more in the distance. I cannot describe the pleasure it gave me every morning to wake up and watch the sun appearing over these snow-covered mountains and I have some excellent photographs to remind me of this view. I also found installed in this hotel two members of the American maritime service who were surveying the quarantine service of Iran and preparing a report to be submitted to the government. The hotel was most comfortable, but extremely expensive at £4/10/0 a night for room alone, and the generous allowance of W.H.O. was hardly sufficient to meet my expenses.

My first task was to contact some of the Iranians and find out who was going to show me round, for that was one of the conditions of service. I decided to walk to the local health department. There I was informed that a conference was in progress but I persuaded the porter to take me up the stairs and I hoped to be able to slip into the room and introduce myself when the meeting was over. However, when I opened the door the first person to fall on my neck was Mr. Sheldon Miller, the American Adminstrator, who had been my right hand when I was with the American Mission in Greece. He was as surprised to see me as I was to see him for, as he said, he had last heard of me after a serious coronary attack which had crippled me! In fact I had had two mild coronary attacks after my return from Greece but had recovered from both. How rumour spreads! That reminded me of the parlour whispering game when a news item was passed round a circle and it was unrecognisable when it reached the last person! Mr. Miller was now a liaison officer between the American Mission and the Iranian Government and spoke the language fluently. Since I had seen him in Greece he had married an Italian girl and had two charming daughters. He had a beutiful temporary home in Teheran. I have already mentioned the way in which he had learned to speak Greek so quickly and now he spoke Persian. He had recently returned from a tour of inspection of Greece and had found that after we had left they had carried out the projects we had suggested.

I found that two persons had been given the task of looking after me whilst in Iran and of taking me round to see what I wanted to see. They were Dr. Zoriassatein, Health Commissioner of Teheran and Director of the Laboratory Service of Iran, and Dr. Mofidi, the acting Director of the Institute of Malariology. The latter was out of the country when I arrived but I was very happy in the care of Dr. Zoriassatein who has remained a very good friend and is still in touch with me.

I had letters of introduction from the Regional Director of W.H.O. to many people including the Chancellor of the University, Dr. Farhad, and Dr. Etemedian, the under-Secretary of the Ministry of

Health. It was pointed out to me that as there was only one faculty at the University, namely medicine, most of the Ministers of the Government were qualified in medicine and some had specialised—this included the Prime Minister, Dr. Eghbad, who, previous to becoming Prime Minister, was the Chancellor of the University of Teheran.

I was taken to meet everybody who could be of help to me including the Prime Minister who regretted that the Shah was in England and would not be back in time for me to be presented. I took careful note of their views and found them all most anxious to do anything in their power to help their country and put it on the map once again. A thousand years had passed since the three great pioneers Rhazes (died 932 A.D.), Haly Ben Abbas (died 994 A.D.) and Avicenna (died 1037 A.D.) had put Persia in the forefront of world medicine and, in the case of Avicenna, of all science in the whole of the world.

Having surveyed Teheran I was glad to break away with Dr. Zoreassatein to travel to Tabris in the north-west of the country, the ancient capital Isfahan and the more modern Shiraz in the south. We had to have passes specially signed by the police authority in order to move about the country and this was arranged by my guide. I found myself in an entirely new world and had to muster my thoughts to note well my strange surroundings. Dr. Zoreassatein was the ideal companion and guide to these cities for he was also Director General of the state laboratories and had therefore visited the cities regularly. All his medical staff looked to Teheran for guidance and instructions. He spoke English perfectly and could therefore act as my interpreter as well.

Tabris could not be said to be rehabilitating very quickly and in that respect was most depressing. It was in Azarbajan, quite near the Caucusses, and had a very mixed population of Turks, Arabs, Armenians Kurds and Russians as well as Persians. It had once been occupied by the Turks and, more recently, at the beginning of the last war, by the Russians. When we visited the city there was a considerable number of Kurds collecting together for their pilgrimage to Mashed, a University town in the north-east of Iran, for they considered it to be almost as high a status to be a "Meshedi" as it was to have been to Mecca. The Kurds are a fine-looking race, spectacularly dressed and carrying long knives in their girdles. They roamed the streets in the evening and a night curfew was in force for the time.

We were met at the little airfield by six doctors who were heads of the different sections of the health services, and not one of whom could speak English. We spent the best part of three days studying the health problems of the city and obtaining the views of the doctors and we paid a visit to a large leper colony for men. A young Persian doctor, wholeheartedly devoted to his work and at great personal sacrifice, was the superintendent and the chief nurses were French monks. They found it very difficult to find staff from Iran and as a last resort they usually appealed to France. That was how they saved a large leper colony of women from having to be closed down in north-east Iran—young French nuns came to the rescue. Similarly the Pasteur Institute in Teheran directed by a charming French doctor prepared vaccines and sera to meet the needs of the country. I was deeply impressed by the great work done in such a quiet and unobtrusive way by the French.

It appeared to me that the doctors I met in Tabris were supervised by their particular individual headquarters in the capital and that they had a feeling of isolation. Before leaving I was taken to see the Governor General who had been Iranian Ambassador in London and spoke English well. We discussed the health problems of the city and I appealed to him to allow each of these doctors to come to him with their problems from time to time and to seek his assistance for dealing with urgent problems. He stood up and shook hands with me and then turned to the doctors and assured them in their own language that they could come and see him at any time. They were all delighted.

There was a handful of British people in Tabris doing very good work. A young doctor from Liverpool had just exposed the source of poisoning which was affecting a number of people in a nearby village, but there appeared to be no dedicated members of a medical school to encourage teaching and research. Even the Dean was a busy medical practitioner and all the other members of the staff were hard at work earning a living. A British nurse was trying with the assistance of a couple more to establish a school of nursing but she had become completely demoralised by conditions and lack of enthusiasm in the city and did not think she could carry on any longer. I met the officer in charge of the British Council and his wife. His health was not good and he was working very hard, teaching English most of his time. He complained bitterly of the many young British "adventurers", often in unfit cars trying to get through to the East. They would boast to the authorities that they had no money and were usually directed by the police to the British Council by mistake, for there was no British Consul in Tabris. More often than not the unfortunate director was out of pocket on the deal and had no hope of reimbursement.

Isfahan, the old capital of Persia, could well have been the most beautiful city in the world, with its bridges, its wonderful mosques and Polo Square where polo was first played in front of the old palace of a former Shah. But, alas, very little of the city had a piped water supply and the infant mortality rate was high.

There were some British people in Isfahan and Bishop Thomson and Mrs. Thomson were much respected throughout the land. They spoke very highly of our present Bishop of St. David's, John Roberts, and his son, who had been out on missionary work. I met a woman doctor who was greatly admired and who did wonderful work in the women's hospital. I discovered that she had been a contemporary of my wife at the Royal Free Hospital in London.

When we arrived at the hotel in Isfahan I found a parcel waiting for me. It was from the director of the British Council who happened to be an old friend of Bristol days. With the parcel was a note—"Herewith a pillow, I have always found the hotel beds very hard on the head." I was most grateful for the loan !

Julfa is a district of Isfahan into which a former Shah compulsorily removed many Armenians from other parts of Iran. It has now the business quarter of the city. There I saw a mosque-type building which in fact is an Armenian Christian Church with pictorial representations of the Bible covering every part of the walls and ceiling. Truly a wonderful sight to behold and some of the paintings were vivid and skilfully painted.

The next city I visited was Shiraz, the beautiful city of the south. In addition to the great memorial tombs to the national poets, Saadi and Hafiz, there were other fine buildings—the University and the new American hospital. These are well worth seeing. However, two other pictures also stand out in my mind. There were some beautiful gardens with fine trees and flowering shrubs and I was told that one of these had been developed by an English resident. The other picture that is still vivid in my memory is that of a medical missionary working in an ancient and antiquated hospital consisting largely of mud buildings. He catered for all classes and when a patient was admitted for an operation or treatment the family was also accommodated in the hospital. He contended that it made for happiness of both patient and family. He would like to have been working as a general practitioner visiting their homes but he could not do as much good in that way. He said that there was a wonderful American hospital built for the rich and the very poor but the "in betweens" could not afford to be ill.

Having visited these four University centres I sat down to consider the people and what I had seen of their mode of life and their institutions. In my mind there was some confusion between the words Persia and Iran for the latter was now the name of the country I was visiting. I learnt that Persia was the old country lying between Isfahan and Shiraz in the centre of Iran which now extends from the Caspian Sea in the north to the Persian Gulf in the south and from Afghanistan in the east to Turkey in the west. It had a population of at least twenty million in 1959. The Persians are concentrated in the middle of the country but there are large numbers of other nationalities on the outskirts. In the north are the Russians, in the west the Turks, Armenians and Kurds and in the south Arabs. To the east and south-east Afghanistans and Pakistanis. The language is Persian of which they are very proud, and this is also spoken in Afghanistan. It is the binding force of the country. Although the language is Persian the alphabet and the script is Arabic, left behind after the Arabs had conquered the country. The people, in particular the Persians, are very proud of their history. Darius and Cyrus made their country famous and in 1961 Persia celebrated the 2,500th anniversary of her monarchy founded by Cyrus the Great whose empire extended from the Indus to the Nile. The remains of their palaces at Persepolis are still worth seeing. Their poets, too, are famous and perhaps the best known to us, but not to the Persians, was Omar Khayyam who was made famous by Fitzgerald's translation of his Rubaiyat. I have already referred to the memorials at Saadi and Hafiz. There are many religions in Iran but the religion of the ruling parties is Mohamedism, the Shiite or the heretic sect of that religion. Attendance at the Mosques is not good but I found the principles of their religion well-entrenched in their homes. Although there are several wonderful mosques in Isfahan there are very few in Teheran. A more recent religion, the Bahai, is making rapid advances in the country. The leader of this sect is living today in America. The Bahais believe that Christ and Mahomet were good prophets and that another, the Bahi in 1850, was another prophet. When he was shot in Tabriz and his body dragged through the streets of that city he became a martyr. His only crime as a very young man

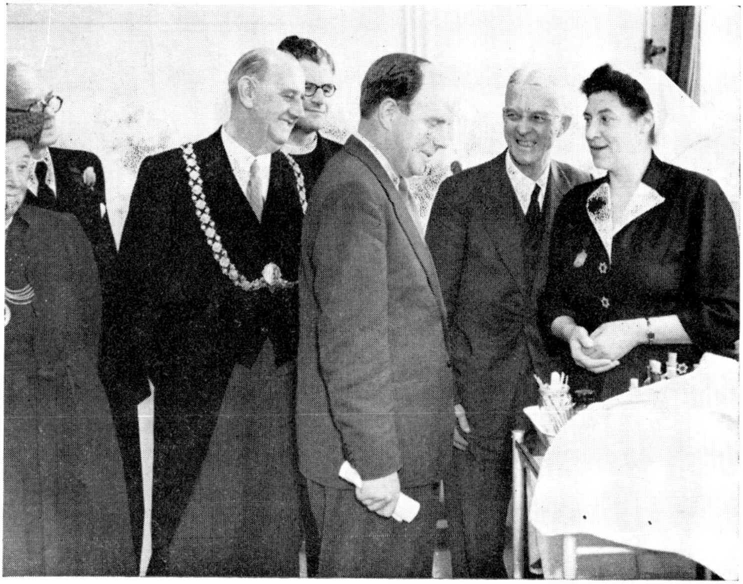

At the official opening of The William Budd Health Centre, Bristol by the Minister of Health in 1952

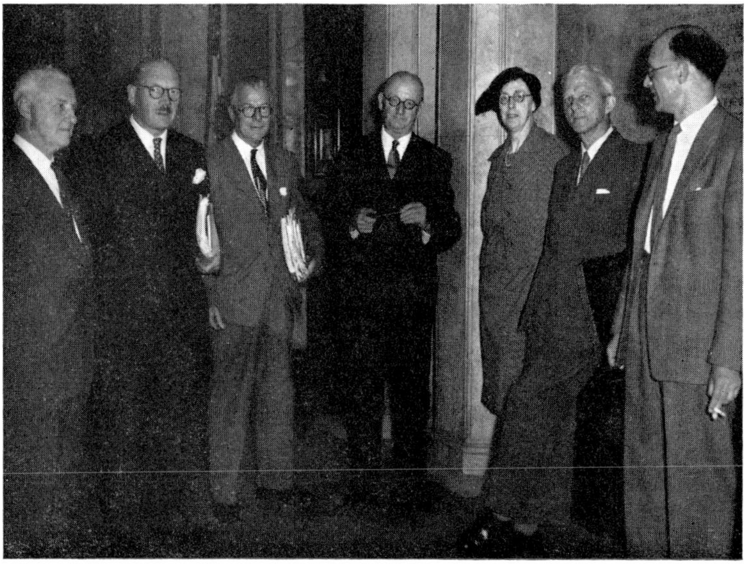

Local Government Commission for England (1960)

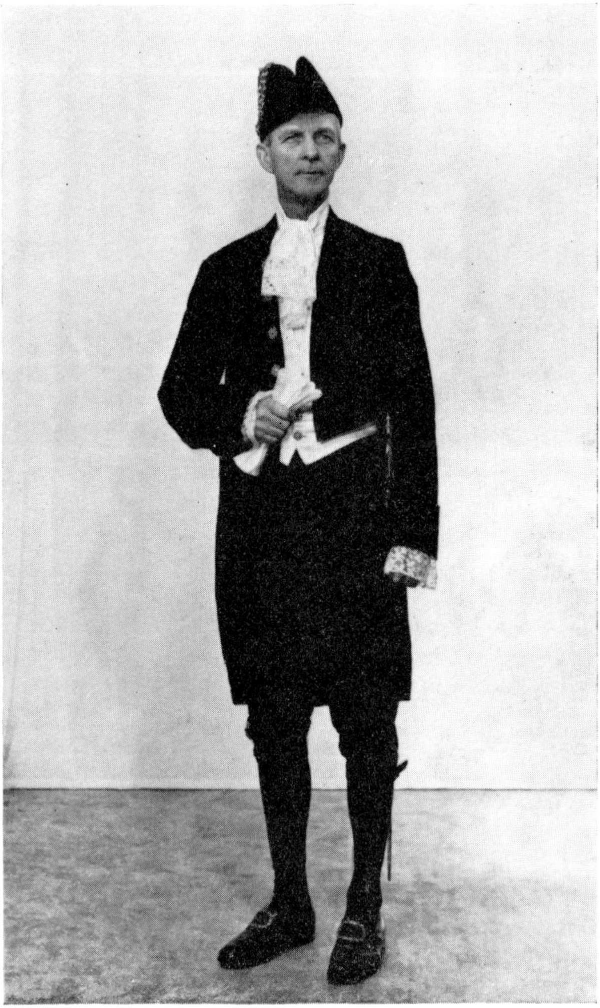

High Sheriff of Caernarvonshire, 1958

in his twenties had been a desire to see honest and straightforward living dominate the life of his fellow countrymen. To this day his life and death are remembered and the number who look back to his good life has increased and is still growing. It is said that all Bahais can be trusted implicity in their dealings. Nevertheless the influence of the Mullah, the Mohamaden priest, is very great. One day the Health Commissioner of Teheran spent an hour strenuously trying to persuade the chief Mullah that it was no sin to inject the human body to cure disease !

There are many wealthy people throughout Iran and especially in Teheran where, at 8,000 ft. they have a town-house and also lovely homes in Shimran another 2,000 ft. higher, where they live in the hot season and where the Shah and the diplomatic corps reside in the summer.

I found a few British contacts who gave me very useful information. For example, the staff of the British Council who were most helpful and doing great work in upholding Britain's good name. But perhaps the most interesting person I met in Teheran was an old English lady, although I hope she never hears that I called her "old" for she was only in her seventies ! She was taking a trip home via the East that summer. She had been the governess to the daughter of the British Ambassador and when her services were no longer required she had started a small private school for young girls. This brought her into contact with many of the influential politicians and others. She told me, at a little private tea party, that she had as many as four or five relatives of the wealthy builder Moussadek, who became Prime Minister and nationalised the oil industry. Most of the British were expelled from the country at that time but she stuck tight. One day a little grand-daughter of Moussadek came to her and said quite firmly that if her grand-dad was going to try and send her from Iran she would take her slipper to him ! The old lady stayed !

After my experience with the American Mission to Greece I found it absolutely necessary to examine the background history of the people and their institutions. I only wish I could have spoken their language before arriving at any conclusions for only in that way is it possible really to know people, to get their confidence and understand their inner thoughts.

When writing my report I had before me four W.H.O. reports written between October 1957 and November 1958 bearing much on the same subject. I felt, however, that they had missed an important point. They had forgotten that they were dealing with a proud people with their own language and that such a nation would not encourage their young people to be taught in a foreign tongue. Indeed, I had a feeling that they did not wish to be "taught" by their visitors but they were open to "suggestions". In Greece in a like manner I imagined them saying "Who the hell are they teaching? Centuries ago when their countries were uncivilised we had Pericles . . ." So the Persians had Cyrus, Darius and Avincenna. I therefore approached my report with these facts in mind. The previous reports had declared against an Institute or at least seemed only half-hearted in its favour. I was whole-heartedly in favour of a Higher Institute whose responsibilities should be not only to train but to register the trained and find them jobs afterwards. It should also review from time to time the progress made in public health and decide priorities for future development. With regard to the language question I herewith quote a paragraph from my report—"In one at least of the reports quoted, mention has been made of the language question. As with many other nations science in recent years has passed by Iran in so far as language is concerned. This creates the difficulty that the country finds itself in at the present time—namely that modern scientific language in which most publications appear, are foreign to Iranians since relatively few Iranians are able to make use of French, English or other languages. For teachers and research-workers this is a matter of extreme importance as indeed it is for people in the same category in all countries. To the rest of the public health-workers, and especially to the field-workers, this becomes a matter of little importance if "in service" training in their own language is kept up to date. What matters most to these field-workers is to be able to understand the people of the community in which they work and to be able to transmit to them knowledge that will enable them to live healthily and happily. In this report, therefore, no suggestions are made regarding the question of the workers learning other languages than Persian. However, it would be most valuable if a translator were employed so that useful reports and pamphlets published in other languages were made available to the field-workers, most of whom have no knowledge of foreign languages. There is little doubt that such a full-time translator could be fully occupied on such work, and should be employed by the 'Institute'." The chief of the Education and Training section in Geneva wrote to say the report had been well received and was a "best-seller".

On our way to Persepolis I was pleased to be able to see some of the nomad tribes going to the mountains with all their belongings. The story of these nomadic tribes and the part they have played in the history of Persia is a thrilling one but not to be told here by me. I was also able to visit a public bath and see the "scrubbers" at work.

I would like to refer to a few other incidents in Iran that have clung to my memory. At a village called Sharria, about fifteen miles from Teheran with a population of about 3,000 there was a demonstration health centre built by the Rockefeller Foundation some years previously. It lacked funds to do the work for which it was intended and it could not obtain the service of trained nurses and doctors. However, it did impress me that such a centre should be included in my report as an outpost of the special Institute for training purposes. Whilst I was visiting this centre the nurse volunteered to show me the inside of a house in the village. After covering her head we entered the house and I had permission to see how man and beast lived together. It was a mud house inside with a special opening down to the "cellar" opposite the front door. In this cavern the goats were packed for the night. On the left, as we entered the house, was the round oven and along the walls of the circular house were alcoves containing the beds and living quarters. I must confess that I had had no picture at the back of my mind as to what a village house in Iran would be like and for that I am glad because the picture I obtained now was a new one and I had no need to destroy any preconceived idea.

I spent several pleasant Sunday afternoons in Dr. Zoriassatein's garden in Shimran eating his luscious cherries. His caretaker-gardener was a tall man with a wife and three young children graded between the ages of seven and three. I have a picture of them taken in the garden and the story Dr. Zoriassatein told me about him is worth repeating as it illustrates a custom of the country. He pointed to the eldest of the three little girls and told me she was the daughter of his gardener's first wife. When she died her husband was very distressed and immediately wrote to her parents living far away in the north-east of the country to tell them of their daughter's death. He asked if they had another daughter old enough to be his wife. If so, would the mother kindly send her measurements so that he might have shirts made for her. In due course he received a reply in the affirmative with pieces of string indicating her measurements. When the shirts were ready he sent for the girl but when she arrived he nearly sent her back. He had been deceived by the measurements sent to him for she was much smaller and younger and only fourteen years old. However, he decided to keep her to look after her sister's baby daughter and then he married her. They had two lovely little girls and she was a wonderful wife, still not quite twenty years old.

One day there was a little procession through the main street of Teheran consisting of two or more hand-trucks with kitchen equipment and little bits of furniture. When I enquired what it was all about I was told it was the bridegroom displaying his possessions before the wedding ceremony.

I met two young English girls in Teheran, one of whom was working for Save the Children Fund and helping to run a home for about four hundred orphans and deserted children. It was a pathetic sight to see the children rushing up to her, they were so excited to see her. It was by no means a model home.

The other was a trained nurse-midwife, having obtained the latter training in our Southmead Hospital in Bristol, although we had not met before. She was now head nurse, or matron, of the maternity training unit which was most highly thought of in all parts of the country.

When we were about to start for Persepolis my guides were asked if they would allow a Lebanese gentleman to come with us. We were very pleased to do so especially as he spoke English and seemed a most pleasant person. Talking to him as we drove along we discovered that he had attended a course of lectures in London and he knew my brother who was at that time Professor of Law and then Vice Chancellor of the University. He made me promise that I would stop for a few days in Beirut as his guest on my way back to Alexandria. The date was arranged but under the circumstances I found it difficult to keep to a programme. Back in Teheran I was asked to give a few lectures at a week-end post-graduate course and this delayed me. A telegram arrived from Beirut—"Expecting you, when are you coming?" Another date was arranged and my promise fulfilled. From Beirut airport I took a taxi to the hotel where Mr. Ghorieb had his office. I was walking along the corridor to reach him when a tall, fine-looking Sudanese appeared walking towards me. He stopped and said "Are you the brother of the Vice Chancellor of London

University ?" "Yes" I replied. "I thought so ; I have been attending his lectures in London. Good day."

When I found Mr. Ghorineb, my Lebanese friend of Persepolis, he immediately spoke on the telephone and I was rushed to see the Minister of Health who was also the Minister of the Interior and held other posts as well. In spite of a queue of people waiting to see him we were shown into his room immediately. Alas, again I knew not his language nor could I carry on well enough in French and he spoke no English. With my friend's help he explained that a cabinet meeting was about to start but would I be good enough to read and comment on a new Health Bill that was coming before Parliament next week. I was then taken to see the senior Medical Officer in charge of the technical side of the scheme. I spent nearly two hours listening to his explanations and when he had finished he asked me if I had any comments or criticism to make. I answered that I had no adverse criticism of the scheme because it was very much like the one I had prepared for Bristol—based on health centres for general practitioners. "Ah" he said, "Bristol, England ?" and when I replied "Yes" he asked me if I knew Abu Shakra. "Yes", I replied, "he was one of my post-graduate students for the Diploma of Public Health". "Well, well, he answered, "he was the doctor who helped us prepare the scheme." Well, what do you know ! as the Americans would say.

That evening Dr. Abu Shakra came to see me and took me out to dinner. It was arranged that I should address a meeting of the doctors about public health matters and try and help them with their problems in this field. It was a most interesting and enthusiastic meeting.

Mr. Ghorieb went out of his way to make my stay a pleasant one. He drove me to see the wonderful ruins at Baalbek and we had lunch at a riverside restaurant where he ordered a bottle of Arak and our table was covered with dishes of "tit-bits" or hors d'oeuvres or what-you-will. When I asked him how many varieties there were he said he thought about forty five. I told him that my wife would never believe me, thinking maybe it was the effect of the Arak ! He said that she must believe me and immediately produced a photographer who took a picture of us and our table which I brought home as evidence—my hair is standing on end but that was due to the breeze in the open air !

I was taken to the plane for Egypt by Mr. Ghorieb next morning and he gave me the address and telephone number of the Minister of

Culture in Cairo and said it would be most interesting for me to contact him.

My wife and I revisited the Lebanon last year with a party arranged under the guidance of Mr. Aslett of the Royal Horticultural Society on a tour to look for plants and visit interesting sites. Again Mr. Ghorieb came to welcome us and arranged for us to meet the chief poet of the country in his home and also a noted historian. It was interesting to learn that an attempt was being made to write Lebanese in Roman script so as to get it more easily understood internationally.

Dr. Abu Shakra, of course, gave us a wonderful welcome to his home and arranged a special dinner to meet his wife, family and friends on the occasion of our forty fourth wedding anniversary. We were given many Lebanese dishes, strange and delicious to us.

At Cairo there was a wait of several hours before the plane for Alexandra would leave. I thought this would be a good opportunity to contact the Minister of Culture as Mr. Ghorieb had suggested. This took a couple of hours and many calls before I finally succeeded in speaking to him. This is where I think I made a mistake and missed an interesting occasion. He wanted me to prolong my stay in Cairo and come and talk to him but I was already feeling guilty because I had 'played truant' in Beirut and I did not wish to involve the World Health Organisation so the meeting did not take place. Whilst I was struggling with the telephone a charming, fine-looking young Egyptian came up to offer his assistance. He was a University graduate and had a brother who was also a graduate. They were both anxious to see a little of the world but could only do so if they could in some way get a scholarship or grant from some country outside Egypt. They were waiting for the young sons of the Vice President of Saudi Arabia who were coming to Cairo to sit an examination. He said their father had been shot by a would-be assassin and had been taken to a London Clinic where he had made a wonderful recovery. He had spoken very highly of the treatment he had received and was determined to adopt some of the customs and ideas he had learned there. In the first place to show more courtesy towards everyone of all ranks and then to try and teach his children and all in his country the importance of depending on oneself rather than expecting help from others. There is certainly need for a good many more clinics of this kind in our own country for our own people !

Soon the time came for me to leave Egypt. I booked by Swiss Air from Cairo but for some reason the plane did not leave that evening and I was their guest at the Sheperd's Hotel for the night. There were no feeding facilities at Sheperd's so that evening I had to cross the street to a luxury hotel and dine in a roof-garden restaurant. The room was very pleasant and seemed to be full of Egyptians but soon, however, a man who I thought might be a Britisher came in and looked around. I had a feeling I had seen him before somewhere so I sent a message by the waiter to invite him to join me at my table and he accepted and made a very entertaining companion. He was the editor of the *American Cotton Journal* and every year went round the world to see his clients in the different countries. His wife usually accompanied him as far as Greece and then returned home. He was interested in the fact that I was Welsh for his only daughter was engaged to a young American of Welsh descent whose chief hobby was buying Welsh books and learning the language. He lived in Memphis Tennessee. Of course, I had to tell him of my "priority call" when I was stranded in Nashville during the war and we came to the conclusion that we had seen each other before. After many guesses we ultimately discovered that we had been staying at the same hotel in Alexandria ! He presented me with a book from the bookstall to read on the plane and I accepted on condition it was a loan which he would come and collect from me in Wales.

One unforgettable incident at Cairo airport was when I was leaving the airport to return to Geneva. I had decided to dispose of all my Egyptian currency before leaving Egypt and had done so, but I still had ten pounds and the equivalent in Swiss francs. I had declared the English pounds on my way out but did not realise that I had not declared the Swiss francs also. The customs official compared the two forms and at once asked where I had obtained the Swiss francs. I was just going to explain when he was called to the telephone. The girl clerk attendant then handed me a clean form which I filled in omitting the Swiss francs. Back came the customs official and said "Where was I ?" The new form was produced, he ticked it and I was passed through. When I reached the other end of the room I beckoned to the girl and said "Thank you very much—that was very sweet of you."

On our flight back to Geneva it was a very clear day and the pilot flew very near to the Matterhorn. I took an excellent photograph of the snowcapped summit whilst a Canadian engineer sitting near me became quite excited and declared that men had been killed trying to get as near as we were to the summit.

Whilst in Iran I was asked several times if I would stay and help establish the Institute but my feelings was that they wanted a younger man who could be moulded more easily into the customs of the country.

CHAPTER X

LOCAL GOVERNMENT COMMISSION FOR ENGLAND 1959—1963

AFTER arriving home a letter came from the chief of medical education and training section at Geneva offering me an appointment in that capacity in South East Asia with headquarters in New Delhi. I would dearly have liked to have taken it but was persuaded, quite rightly, that at my age it was not easy for the human body to acclimatize. I had had evidence of this when, after my refusal, another medical officer from Scotland had undertaken a tour of Nigeria, before that country had Independence, for the Colonial Office and he died shortly afterwards. It is one of the ironic truths that when a man is young and physically fit to undertake appointments of this kind he lacks experience and knowledge. When he has acquired these qualifications he is too old to undertake these tasks without risk to his health.

When I arrived hom from Geneva in 1959 there was a letter awaiting me. It was from Sir Henry Hancock, the Chairman of the Local Government Commission for England. He wanted to know if I would be interested to join the Commission and if so would I come up to London to see him and talk it over. Now I had been so busy with my own personal programme that I had read little about this new Commission and my passing thought was that it would go the way of all Commissions if it clashed with politics ! However, all my life I had been concerned directly or indirectly with local government and I was just getting it "out of my blood" when lo ! here it came again. It was agreed that I should join and I received my Royal warrant, signed by Princess Margaret in the absence of the Queen.

It is not generally realised that administration of central government departments differs from that of local authorities. In the former the chief permanent official is an administrator and a person with good general knowledge, particularly of the classics and history. He usually has experts to advise him on the technologicaal problems with which his department is involved. He, however, is completely responsible for the administration and for advising the Minister who is the "Big Chief". This did not always work too well. When Sir Arthur Newsholme was chief Medical Officer to the (central) local government board, which later became the Ministry of Health, he revealed, after his retirement, that some of his reports concerning health, or more accurately disease, were pigeon-holed and never saw the light of day. No doubt there is much relaxation in this latter since those days, but even so no technically (Scientifically !) qualified officer, or so I believe, is known to have been appointed chief of a central government department in which he is an expert. An exception is in the general Post Office where an engineer may be in command. The arguments in favour of such a course that is not appointing an expert—are powerful. It is all a question of money and there must not be a person in charge with a "bee in his bonnet", i.e. a specialist. He could, of course, be a cricketer or a golfer or even a poet. Besides the "Treasury", that unknown, veiled power behind closed doors could not possibly deal with a flock of technicians from different departments ! They must be able to speak the same civil service language as themelves.

In local government, on the other hand, the chief of the department is usually a technical officer, a doctor, an architect, an education officer and so on, all trained and qualified in the particular branch of knowledge they are expected to administer in the field. The Town Clerk is their legal adviser and co-ordinator and advises the Council and its committees but does not interfere in the departmental administration.

The Local Government Commission was not concerned with central government administration although the facts stated had to be borne in mind. They certainly were concerned with local government administration. It was most noticeable that a competent, tactful chief officer could get the approval of his council more readily to the expenditure of money and so to the development of his particular service. Even with the same authority there was great disparity in the proportion of its financial resources allotted to the different departments. In regard to some of these it was difficult to diagnose the cause of their failure. Could it be the fault of the officer—his ability, his approach to the problem or his relation to the committee and more especially to the chairman ? Could the fault be with the committee through their interference with administrative details, especially by the chairman which it is known only too well can demoralise any chief officer. The officer cannot afford to alienate his committee and so he swims with the tide. If there is one reform that is urgently required it is to make the chief officer responsible in the public eye for his success or failure and to detach committees and councillors from administrative functions. Their responsibilities lie in obtaining for the people they represent the services and amenities they want and for which they pay. The active details of carrying out these services must be left to the expert.

But this was not for discussion in our Commission. Our terms of reference were very limited. We were concerned with creating proper boundaries for effective county and county borough units. This was useful work if it could be carried out, but every member of every local authority would know what was good for the other area whilst "We are all right as we are" was the cry that I expected.

We had to stand by one principle—that nothing could be achieved by criticising the existing local authorities, however bad their service might be. It was important to stress the changing world and the increasing responsibilities to be cast on local administration in the future. This would cost a good deal more money—more than many could afford—so what could they do about it?

Having brooded on these matters for so many years I was agreeably surprised to see the open-minded way in which the seven members of the Commission approached the subject. As we delved into the problems of the multifarious duties the local authorities had to perform we were amazed that such reasonable services were provided by such clumsy, illogical and irrational organisations. We realised that small, compact and poor units often had their merits no less than the large, wealthy remote ones, but of differing value to the community. Similarly their weaknesses were most apparent. Now our problem was how to mould a unit locally that would retain the merit and lose some, at least, if not all, of its weakness. There was a further complication, so well known to most of us, that the different services had their own problems in relation to size and financial resources. We were not expected to find the best unit locally for a particular service but for all of them as they existed.

It was quite apparent that our terms of reference were too narrow but at the same time we could propose improvements which could lead to the next step in progress. In this spirit we proceeded to survey England. We travelled far and wide and some of our recommendations were accepted by Parliament such as the City of Teeside, the reorganisation of the Black Country and many minor alterations. However I have no intention of pursuing this subject. It is far too complicated for this little effort in reminiscing.

After more than four years I found the travelling about, with many nights away from home and a complete change of habits, at my late stage of life a little too strenuous and when the time came for re-appointment I specially requested that my name should not be included. The experience merely confirmed my views and fears. Local authorities vary immensely in their efficiency throughout the land—and it is not lack of financial resources alone that is responsible. We knew after inspecting a service where there was an efficient or inefficient Chief Officer and a helpful or obstructive authority, and especially when each was playing its own part. A few interviews usually gave us the clue but it would be difficult for any reorganisation to solve all these problems.

CHAPTER XI

REFLECTIONS

WHEN we acquired our small farm we thought it would be great fun and an occupation to have some poultry and a small herd of Jersey cows. Through the kindness of the Professor of Veterinary Surgery at Bristol I bought eight Jersey heifers from well-known breeders in Jersey. They were lovely little creatures and, after a time, the eight came into milk. However, after a year or two one full-time worker did not appear to be quite sufficient to cover the work for a full week. The man had to have his half-days and some week-ends off duty and the climax came one Saturday afternoon when he was off and my wife proceeded to the dairy and I to the cowshed to do the milking. There was an electricity failure and the eight heifers had to be milked by hand which was a new experience to all of them and some of them did not take kindly to it. It was as well that my early training on the farm had prepared me for such an emergency but I did find it a good deal more trying and tiring than it had seemed to be during my school-days at home. With some six hundred hens to be cared for in deep litter and young chicks to rear the work gradually became a labour and no longer a pleasure. Then I was called away to an assignment with World Health, and so, to our great sorrow, we had to bring our farming adventure to an end.

When I finally retired from active service in 1964 I was hoping to realise my wish to sit and "meditate" ' under the cherry tree '. That lovely old farmhouse and ten acres in Criccieth and my companion of forty years were waiting for me to settle down. All the children had settled their future careers and decided to establish their own homes. They were old enough to look after themselves and yet these homes and the new arrivals into them gave us much anxiety as well as interest and pleasure. The grandchildren are now growing up and we see our own children facing the same problems that we had to tackle. Thirteen years have passed since I expressed my views in writing, in addresses in the United States and published in *The Medical Officer,* October 1952, and these years have made no difference to the type or size of the problems—unless maybe they have somewhat increased the difficulties. I quote from that article :—

"One of the most difficult tasks I have ever undertaken is to bring up a family of four children. As you know, who have been in the same position, the danger is not neglect but to know how much help ought to be given, when the child starts to walk, starts to talk, when he goes to school and certainly when he sits examinations and when he starts courting. How much should we interfere? And what a blow it is when we realise that they want a home of their own and can do without us. We would like to put the benefit of our experience and advice at their disposal but do they either need it or want it? And so it goes on from generation to generation. Ten years ago the families of Britain joined together to form a welfare state. It was the wish of the vast majority of the people however much it may be criticised from inside or out."

In Britain the State is trying to bring up its children. We are studying our problems, our children and our families. How much help ought we to give them? Are we giving them too much or should we give give them more? How much protection do they want and how much can they do for themselves? These are very difficult questions to answer and we are, as usual, trying to muddle through and find the best way of settling these problems. Of course, under certain circumstances, too much can be given. Nevertheless, it is perhaps better that a few should be spoiled by too much help than that any should suffer from the lack of it. Yet note this story from *The Facts of Fiction* by Norman Collins concerning Dr. Samuel Johnson :—

"It is one of the pieces of good fortune of literary history that we possess so exact an account of the fantastic events that led to the publication of *Rasselas*. Towards the end of January 1759 Dr. Johnson's mother died and Johnson, in his usual condition of urgent insolvency, had to pay the expenses of the funeral as well as other outstanding debts. With the sublime confidence which was his he wrote *Rasselas*. He sat down in his Gough Square garret and in the evenings of one week sent it to the press in portions as it was written and did not take the trouble to read it till he revised it for a second edition. Doddsley paid him altogether £125 for it, enough to bury a whole family . . . Three months later *Rasselas* was published. Dr. Johnson was temporarily solvent again and the cruel system that puts genius to the treadmill was once more vindicated. *Rasselas* is indeed one of the best answers today to the "pensions for poets" kind of talk that not infrequently breaks out. A mind like Dr. Johnson's is rare, but sloth such as Dr. Johnson's is common and Johnson was an author who worked with zest only when the bailiffs of fate were greedily pressing for an early settlement of accounts . . ."

As a member of the older generation I have seen too much discipline exercised both by parents and by the authorities. The Church, from whom forgiveness would be expected, is even today in some matters unforgiving. Not long ago, as evidenced by looking at tombstones in some of our cemeteries, young men were hanged for stealing sheep. Of course, there was bound to be a reaction. Today, however, we have to contend with a "permissive society", some of whom say they believe in "absolute freedom," whatever that may mean. And yet nature itself is far from being "permissive". Transgress its laws and you will be punished without a doubt. Excesses and deficiencies of various kinds equally are risks to health, even where the necessities of life are involved. Too much food is as harmful as too little, too much or too little drink likewise, and nowadays it is thought that too little exercise is as likely as too much exercise to cause heart disease. The Greeks called the safety line "the golden mean". This requires discipline—self-discipline where our own welfare is concerned, and discipline by the government to maintain a healthy community. Of course, it must be reasonable and firm, for these are conditions against reactions. In a growing, young community as much as with the growing child punishment and reward are important signposts of the direction he has to travel.

After giving up farming we turned our attention to gardening which was not quite so exhausting but equally interesting and rewarding, although not financially, I may add ! There was very little evidence of an old garden in the wilderness of weeds and brambles we found around the house but there were many large stones, probably from the ruins of part of the old house, and these formed the basis of a rock garden. The house stood surrounded by small fields so we were able to push out the boundaries of the garden. We soon realised that our horticultural knowledge was somewhat limited so we joined the Royal Horticultural Society and visited many gardens and nurseries for ideas and advice, including the famous gardens at Wisley and the Saville Gardens in Windsor Park. We also joined the French Horticultural Society and spent a week in Paris touring the gardens of the Ile de France with a party of French gardening enthusiasts. In spite of language difficulties we enjoyed this experience immensely. Most of the gardens we visited belonged to Chateaux and were laid out in the grand manner with lakes and fountains, lawns, long avenues of trees and hedges and statuary. We visited a famous rose garden where we were taken through a long path showing the history of the rose starting with the wild-rose at one end and finishing at the other end with bushes of the latest varieties under cultivation. No doubt we were prejudiced but the so-called "English garden" we visited belonging to a wealthy French family living a few miles from Paris appealed to us much more than the vast gardens of the Chateaux.

The following year, in April, we joined a party of twenty plant-hunting enthusiasts on a tour of the Lebanon under the guidance of Mr. Ken Aslet who is in charge of the rock gardens at Wisley. His wife accompanied him and acted as a very efficient and charming guide rounding up stragglers and generally looking after our comforts and the smooth running of the expedition. We flew to Beirut where we stayed for five days. An excellent Lebanese driver took us by bus on a daily excursion to a different place each day within a radius of about thirty miles either along the coast or up one of the valleys into the foothills. Our first day we went to Byblos passing many small plantations of lemons, oranges and loquarts in full bloom and their perfume was quite heavy. We had not seen or tasted loquarts before. They look like small apricots in bunches of four or five and each contains two or three large almond-like seeds. We brought several seeds back with us and planted them in our cool greenhouse—a few germinated and we now have two small trees which we have planted in sheltered positions in the garden but it is doubtful whether we shall ever see any fruit. At Sidon, after visiting the ancient fort we entered the old courtyard surrounded by tall buildings that used to be a "caravanserai" where the merchants put up for the night and the gates were shut and barred against robbers. The buildings were festooned with bouganvillia and bright with geraniums in every balcony. In the centre of the courtyard was a small grove of lemon and orange trees.

After five days in Beirut we drove to The Cedars—a remarkable journey from seal level to seven thousand feet in a few hours along steep winding roads. In the picturesque villages clinging to the hillside where we often stopped to explore, every house seemed to have its own small patch of hillside on which they had terraced the land and grew vines and apple trees. At the Cedars we were above the snow line and there were still a few late skiers on the slopes above the hotel where we stayed for three nights. The next few days were very sunny and the snow was melting rapidly. It was surprising to see the masses of anemones and cranesbill pushing their way through the ground wherever the snow had melted. The cedar forests have been reduced to small clumps of trees by indiscriminate felling for timber but the Lebanese government has now established a forestry undertaking and they have nurseries of small trees with which they are afforesting the slopes once more.

Our last few days were spent at Chtaura, about two thousand feet up in the hills behind Beirut on the Damascus road. We travelled towards Damascus to see the ruins of the ancient Temples at Baalbek and along the fertile plain of Anjar, part of Old Canaan. We passed through many miles of vineyards and good pasture land and saw the black tents of the Bedouins who were camping with their camels, usually on uncultivated land. This is apparently a custom or benefit both to the farmer and the Bedouins for the farmer gets cheap labour and the camels help to manure the soil. As soon as the patch has been cultivated the Bedouins move on.

We had been warned to apply for a permit from the Ministry of Agriculture and Fisheries to bring back plants to this country and this we did. I now have a small corner of the garden in which some of our Lebanese plants are thriving.

In my new occupation I am dealing with a stable community of living things. Perforce plants are tied down to earth which is more than can be said of human beings. Yet I doubt if they are more predictable in early life in their behaviour than men and women at that stage. Like humans they also would be all right if they were not interfered with by outside agencies ! There is one common factor—life. When I went to the university first, over fifty six years ago I listened to Professor H. J. Fleure describing "life" and trying to explain it. It was most impressive and made me think. How very important such talks can be to influence young people.

Since taking up gardening seriously I have been most impressed by the response of living plants to their environment. Like animals, including man, they prepare for the seasons. Some cast off their sensitive parts and go to sleep, others merely cut down their activities and brace themselves, by hardening, to meet the strain of winter. They respond carefully to temperature, moisture and food. But in particular one eucalyptus tree has amazed me. It was about eighteen inches tall when it was planted but within three years it has grown to ten feet. During those three years, however, about six inches of the top was killed by frost during each winter and this is where the strange behaviour showed itself. When the cold season was over and growth was beginning I could imagine the "brain headquarters" of the tree sending out a message to the two topmost side branches that damage had been done to the leader. Following this they would grow at a rapid pace, but for some reason or other one of them grows quicker and straighter and henceforth becomes the "leader". This kind of behaviour in an animal would be called instinct. What it is called in a plant I do not know, nor does it matter for it is but a name. In truth it is intelligent behaviour in response to its environment and is characteristic of life in any shape or form. From time to time I have to transplant shrubs and even small trees because they dislike exposure to the weather or maybe being sheltered too much. Sometimes they even do not like their neighbours ! How little we really know about life.

My little grandson was surprised to hear some one calling me doctor one day. He came back to me and said "Taid (Grandpa) I did not know you were a doctor". "Didn't you my boy ?" "No, I thought you were a gardener." "Thank you very much—that is what I have been aiming at for several years and you are the first to pay me the compliment."

And now my chief attention is directed to watching growing plants, with maybe an occasional glance over my shoulder at the old problems and their new "solvers".

In the seventy years I have seen many changes. It is easy to compare certain aspects of life in the country in those early days with those of today. Then there were plenty of horses with dust and flies about but very few motor cars and no fumes. Flying was considered to be the hobby of cranks and had no effect in drowning the bleating of the sheep, the lowing of cattle and the songs of the birds, whereas today men and women in some parts of the country cannot sleep in peace for the sound of aeroplanes. The computer and the automatic man (robots) were subjects for horror fiction—far from reality. Yet now, with the help of these instruments, men have visited and walked on the moon.

I wonder what all these changes will mean to the individual and to his social life ? Midst the loud noises created by protesters it is difficult to hear the voices of thinking people. We hear and talk about democracy, government, community and organisations of all kinds but I believe Austin Freeman is right when he said :—"The destiny of the race will be determined not by the wealth of accumulated knowledge but by the quality of the individuals of which the race is composed."